Three Paths of Devotion

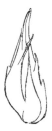

Three Paths of Devotion:
Goddess, God, Guru

by

Prem Prakash

Yes International Publishers
Saint Paul, Minnesota

For information and permissions address:

Yes International Publishers
1317 Summit Avenue
Saint Paul, MN 55105-2602
Telephone: 651-645-6808
www.yespublishers.com

Library of Congress Cataloging-in-Publication Data

Prem Prakash, 1959-
Three paths of devotion / Prem Prakash.
   p. cm.
ISBN 0-936663-27-8
1. Yoga, Bhakti. 2. Spiritual life—Hinduism. I. Kshemaraja, 11th
cent. Pratyabhijna Hridayam. II. Shankara. Nirvanashatktam. III.
Tulasidas, 1532-1623. Hanuman Chalisa. IV. Title.
BL 1238.56.B53 P74 2002
294.5'436—dc21
                                                2002006748

Printed in the United States of America

Dedication

I offer this book
at the feet of the
One
who loves to love,
and to those
who serve that love.

Contents

Acknowledgements

I offer my great appreciation to Theresa King of Yes International Publishers, who has worked with much dedication and devotion to bring about this book.

I'd also like to thank my dear wife, Lesley Ambika Gibbs, for her inspiration and help during the writing and editing of this book.

I also thank the *satsang* of the Green Mountain School of Yoga, particularly those who have taken vows of spiritual friendship with me—James Ashenfelter, John Small, Joe Langerfeld, and Joshua Cooper—for their enthusiasm and support.

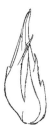

Introduction

To wake one morning and find an unannounced gift on your doorstep that could change your life forever would hardly be expected, especially before breakfast! This book was just such a gift early one day.

For those of us in Western culture who seek self-realization in our lifetime, Prem Prakash's engaging scriptural translations and acute comments opens an ancient vista that ignites our curiosity and challenges our current paradigms on spiritual destiny.

Thanks to his exceedingly readable renditions, the reader embarks upon a vibrant tour de force that sparks human intelligence in ways that would make Plato's devotees and Aristotle's peripatetic followers envious. Who would even suspect that enfolded in those opening twenty verses of the Heart of Self-Realization is what Western theologians might call a transcendental theology? Theologians and philosophers attempt, through their various sciences, to render the ultimate explanation to the entire universe. The hitch is that they do it from their point of view.

This is not to demean their sincere efforts to uncover the truth of things, but our doorstep has yielded something more astonishing. This tiny treatise purports to be from God's point of view. And she has got quite a vision! In fact, it is an infinite one, a never-ending creative evolution and devolution in which she expresses her delight with her inherent wisdom. The bonus is that she shares it with her family—the multifarious creatures that continually emerge and inhabit the planets in her field of manifestation. The Mother in her historic roles, for example, plays Gepetto, whose unalloyed love brings us into being. She is the Pied Piper whose celestial sounds dances us into the garden of enchantment, our remembrance of who we truly are. This treatise closes the abyss between the divine and the human that so discourages humankind in its hours of tragedy.

Awash in misinformation regarding the nature of what is real and our place in this reality, we gather up the second gem on our doorstep consisting of six very compacted verses. Here philosophers will discover one of their own, a traveler of life named Shankara. For one who seeks the unity in the diversity, who immediately wants to cut to the chase, whose intelligence prefers only the metaphysical heights, these lean, scintillating verses are made for you. A word of caution for Western pursuers of ultimacy: Shankara is not for timid speculators.

The final gem upon our doorstep has an unusual brilliance that induces all sorts of practical ideas. Opening it up we meet a perennial story for our tragic times in the third millennium. We ask for leaders and pray to the gods of various religions for solace, safety, and protection. In our reflective moments, we yearn for healing, for wholeness, not just for ourselves but for the peoples at large. We recognize that our individualism can't exclude others; we want to travel our path with friendship. Yet we hesitate to give our hearts for lack of trust. Who can resist allegiance, fidelity, commitment, and devotion when offered without strings attached? Can we rise to the standing invitation when it is offered? In these forty verses we are granted a profound glimpse into the esoteric significance of the unity of friendship, the human and the divine as played out in the roles of disciple and guru.

Classical Yoga asserts that awareness fosters freedom. In these three masterpieces, one learns that there is a devotional awareness of the heart waiting to be found. There one finds a companion for eternity.

Swami Jaidev Bharati
(Justin O'Brien, M.A., Drs.Th., D.Ph.)

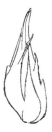

Preface

In the yogic tradition, an aspirant is free to worship any image of God which provides inspiration. The yogi makes personal the relationship with the Divine Being by envisioning divinity in a form that one can love and appreciate. This form is called an *Ishtadeva,* a "chosen deity."

The concept of *Ishtadeva,* of a personally chosen form of God, may be difficult for many Westerners to appreciate. Our Judeo-Christian culture presents a myth which purports very dictatorially that there is only one true image of God—that of the stern but somehow loving Father. We have also been told that creating images of God is idolatrous, with some societally approved exceptions such as Christmas displays.

This myth is culturally prejudiced, and is revealed as such when seen in the light of many of the world's religions, particularly those of India. In India, the devout feel free to worship any of literally thousands of images of Gods and Goddesses. Each individual is welcome to choose a form attractive to him or her. It is even said light-heartedly that there exists a different form of God for each Hindu. But monotheism simply means there is only one God; it does not mean that God will appear to all people in the same way.

In this book, I present three of the primary forms of God long worshipped by yogis. These are: the Immanent Goddess, the Transcendent God, and the Guru. I have chosen three texts which describe the depth and beauty of each of these *Ishtadeva.* In the texts, I have translated the original Sanskrit into English and, as is traditional, I have offered a commentary on each of the verses. I hope my commentary brings to life the vitality of the traditions being presented, and also helps the reader understand how brilliantly the yogic tradition uses myth and symbols to convey to the nature of the Divine Being.

Prem Prakash

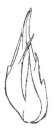

Part I

The Immanent Goddess

This book will begin with the Goddess, or Divine Mother, because she is the origin and culmination of all existence. She is the one that gives birth to the universe, the power which sustains life, and the force of transformation we call death. She is the Alpha and Omega of all.

The text I have selected to represent the Goddess is the *Pratyabhijna Hridayam,* "The Heart of Self-Realization," a true masterpiece of spiritual literature. In only 20 short verses, its author, Kshemaraja, conveys the essence of a sublime philosophy, cosmology, ontology, and spiritual path. He discusses the nature of the Goddess, how the universe manifests, the constitution of individual consciousness, and how the individual can yoke his or her consciousness to the divine. Although we have no historical information on Kshemaraja, scholars have placed his writings in the 10th century.

The *Pratyabhijna Hridayam* is intended as a distillation of the essential teachings of the *Pratyabhijna* system. The term *pratyabhijna* means "Self-realization," but it also implies a certain recognition, or remembering. The individual soul has forgotten its true identity as having arisen from the Goddess. The nature of this forgetfulness will be outlined in the text, as well as in ways which aspirants may attain enlightenment, that is, remembering their divine heritage.

In order to fully appreciate the *Pratyabhijna Hridayam,* it will be helpful for the reader to understand something of the creation myth underlying its philosophy. The Divine Mother, also called the Goddess of Universal Consciousness, holds the embryo of the universe in her womb. She gives birth to the entire cosmos, with infinite galaxies, solar systems, and sentient beings of various forms. It is said that in our world alone there are 8,400,000 different forms in which sentience can manifest. But the Mother does not care to simply bear children. She also wishes to nurture them so they can fulfill their divine potential of being playmates and dancers in her cosmic game. She does this by creating worlds in which individual souls can learn lessons of wisdom and compassion. The nature of the Mother's work is one of the most significant features of the *Pratyabhijna Hridayam* and will be discussed in detail in the text and commentary.

One more point needs to be made about the joy which drives the Mother to create, sustain and eventually reabsorb the universe back into herself. This joy is, in the ultimate sense of the word, ecstatic. For most of us, joy is thought of as being an increase in our level of happiness, and ecstasy as somehow being that same joy at an even higher level. Something like parlaying $10 at a gambling table into $100, then into $1000.

Our experiences of personal happiness fall short, however, of the bliss that awaits us when we transcend the personal and fall into the Divine. For the joy of the Mother is maddeningly intense. It is orgasmic, a wild force which overpowers all other concerns and considerations. All limited experiences pale before her dance of untamed abandon. She brings her devotees into a universe filled with throbbing bliss. She shows the yogi the vision of creation as her cosmic dance hall.

Pratyabhijna Hridayam
The Heart of Self-Realization
by
Kshemaraja

1

चितिः स्वतन्त्रा विश्वसिद्धिहेतुः ॥

citiḥ svatantrā viśvasiddhihetuḥ

*The Goddess of Universal Consciousness,
flowing with unfettered freedom,
displays her awesome power
in the manifestation of the universe.*

The *Pratyabhijna Hridayam* opens by introducing the Goddess and her potency. Inherent in her Universal Consciousness is the sublime urge to create the universe. This creative impulse is not the result of any external prompting, limited desire, nor even purpose. It is a demonstration of her own unbridled freedom. Being full and complete, she chooses to bring forth a universe of limitation and incompletion.

Theologians and philosophers have debated for centuries why God created the world, and they have postulated virtually every possible theory. This is not necessarily problematic, and the topic of philosophical differences is addressed in verse 8 of this text. Beyond the reach of ideas and speculations, however, live the great yogis like Kshemaraja, who have realized the truth. From their vantage point, they see the Goddess has no reason for creating the world. It is simply her nature to pour forth universes in divine creative expression.

The yogis tell us there is no purpose to creation because purpose is an invention of the human mind. We see purpose because we desire our lives to be purposeful. This is well and good, but it leaves us short of realizing the bliss of creation. For the Divine Mother, there can be no purpose because she is eternally complete and whole, filled with the utmost satisfaction and joy. Her play of creation is like an endless spring of happiness and pure creativity, gushing forth and overflowing all containers. She expresses her unlimited love by creating the limited, and then filling it with the love from which it was produced.

The universe is a masterpiece, it is the demonstration of the Mother's artistry. The absolute Godhead is transcendent to creation as the masculine principle, Shiva. But the Goddess, the Divine Mother, the feminine principal, is entirely immanent in creation. The will and joy of the Goddess causes waves of forms and sentient beings to arise from the ocean of her being. Such is her primal, fantastic delight.

2

स्वेच्छया स्वभित्तौ विश्वमुन्मीलयति ॥

svecchayā svabhittau viśvamunmīlayati

By her own will,
she unfolds the universe
on the screen of herself.

The Divine Mother is both the efficient cause and the material cause of creation. She is the Goddess of Creation and also exists as creation. She does not rule her creation from afar; she inhabits everything with her consciousness. She is everyone and everything. The contemporary saint, Shree Maa of Kamakhya has said, "The God you seek is present in every atom of creation."

The Goddess abides in all of creation without losing her identity of being its Mother. In a beautiful paradox, creation is the total expression of all her energy, yet she remains full and complete. No material analogy can be applied, for she transcends the laws of physics which dictate that when energy is expounded a cause is lessened by the creation of effects.

In addition to the role of creator, the Goddess of Universal Consciousness is the preserver and destroyer. As preserver, she maintains the balance between growth and decay which enables the world to exist. As destroyer, she is constantly transforming existence into ever new forms.

In the mythology of the tantric systems, of which this *Pratyabhijna Hridayam* forms a part, the cycle of birth, death, and rebirth is seen as the dance of the Goddess. When an aspirant attains this realization, he or she takes a place in the divine dance. The world does not change, but one's perception of the world changes. All things are seen as expressions of the Mother's creative abandon. All sounds are notes in her cosmic jam session and all movement is her dance.

3

तन्नाना अनुरूपग्राह्यग्राहकभेदात् ॥

tannānā anurūpagrāhyagrāhakabhedāt

The universe appears diverse
as a result of the different
ways that individual subjects
perceive and interact with objects.

This verse explains the reason why the one universe appears differently to various beings. Species experience the universe differently because they are endowed with different mechanisms of communication with the external world. The difference in the structure of the brain and senses provides varying capacities for interaction with the world. A dog, for example, can hear sounds that the human ear cannot, but our canine friends cannot see the variety of colors available to the human eye.

A healthy human being has five *jnana indriyas,* receptive sensory organs. These are the eyes, nose, tongue, ears, and skin, by which a person can see, smell, taste, hear, and touch. There also exist five *karma indriyas,* active sensory organs. These are the hands, feet, tongue, anus, and reproductive organs, by which an individual may grasp, approach, speak, excrete, and reproduce. The processes of the *indriyas* are coordinated by the lower mind, called *manas. Manas* is essentially a computer which processes the incredible array of sensory data, and coordinates it into a composite picture of the outside world. *Manas* is overseen by the *buddhi,* the intellect, which makes decisions and directs activity.

The mind and *indriyas* influence the way the world is perceived and interacted with, but they do so on only one level of reality, the physical world. Yogic cosmology describes seven levels of reality. They are:

1. *Satya Loka*—The realm of eternal truth, wherein dwells Shiva and the Goddess in eternal love.

2. *Tapa Loka*— The realm of illumination, wherein dwells God as the supreme guru, the root teacher of all spiritual traditions.

3. *Jnana Loka*—The realm of wisdom, wherein dwell individualized souls aware of their unity in diversity.

4. *Mahar Loka*—The realm of the great creation, wherein dwell the beings who are influenced by the great illusion of individuality.

5. *Swar Loka*—The realm of thought, wherein live beings who identify with the functions of their mental apparatus.

6. *Bhuvar Loka*—The realm of feelings, wherein live beings who identify with their emotional responses.

7. *Bhu Loka*—The realm of matter, wherein live beings who identify with their physical bodies.

The identity of a sentient being is the result of awareness situated on one of these seven levels of reality. Most human beings dwell in the realms of *bhu, bhuvar,* and *swar.* Only those who have identified with their reality as spiritual beings are able to access the realms above *swar.*

All species of life on our planet are to be respected, but human being are uniquely valuable for two reasons. The first is that they are the only ones endowed with the full capacity of the *buddhi.* Other life-forms are capable of feeling emotions and elementary thought, but only the *buddhi* of the human being is capable of engaging in meta-thought, thinking about thinking. Humanity is the only species capable of forming a science of psychology, the study of the psyche.

The second reason that humanity holds a unique and significant place in the planetary scheme is that the human body holds within it a subtle structure of seven *chakras,* or energy centers, which are coordinated with the seven levels of macrocosmic reality. These centers are not physiological structures, though they have physical coordinates in the glands.

These seven centers are:

1. *Sahasrara Chakra*—The center located at the crown of the head, related to *satya loka* and the attainment of absolute enlightenment by a human being.

2. *Ajna Chakra*—Located behind and between the eyebrows, related to the pineal and pituitary glands as well as the *tapa loka,* is also known as "the third eye," the seat of the inner guru and the attainment of enlightenment.

3. *Vishuddha Chakra*—Located behind the throat, related to the thyroid gland and the *jnana loka,* this chakra influences higher creativity and communication.

4. *Anahata Chakra*—Located behind the center of the chest and related to the *mahar loka,* this chakra is related to compassion.

5. *Manipura Chakra*—Located behind the solar plexus and related to the *swar loka,* this chakra is associated with personal power and issues of security.

6. *Svadhishthana Chakra*—Located behind the genitals and related to the *bhuvar loka,* this chakra is associated with reproduction and issues of pleasure.

7. *Muladhara Chakra*—Located the base of the spine and related to the *bhu loka*, this chakra is associated with the root of individual existence and the fear of egoic death.

While every human being is endowed with each of these *chakras,* the activation of the chakras comes about as a result of spiritual development. For most, the higher chakras exist in only their dormant state, as potentials. Still, the mere notion that these aspects of consciousness remain latent in every human being is cause for respect and service to all.

4

चितिसंकोचात्मा चेतनोऽपि संकुचितविश्वमयः ॥

citisaṁkocātmā cetano'pi saṁkucitaviśvamayaḥ

By an act of Self-limitation,
the Goddess of Universal Consciousness
sacrifices her infinite awareness
and becomes the individual soul.
Correspondingly, her experience of the universal
is now limited to that
of a body/mind complex.

This verse serves to amplify and further explain the principals described in the previous verse. It is the Goddess alone who abides in all beings. It is her consciousness which gives rise to all sentience. She does this through an act of *yajna,* sacrifice or offering. This sacrifice is the giving of herself to all life, by which form is created and animated. The origination of individual souls begins with *yajna,* and *yajna* is the primary principal of harmony throughout the universe.

The Goddess performs her offering, the primal sacrifice, through a process of giving herself away into the worlds she has created. The Vaishnavas say that God creates the world in three stages. First, God creates myriads of universes which exist like bubbles floating in eternal, infinite cosmic space. God then divides each universe/bubble into three spheres: the physical, the astral, and the heavenly. In the final stage of creation, God enters into each universe, animating dull matter with life force and sentience.

Herein lies the solution to the great debate of Creationism versus Darwinian Evolution. Creation is a divine act, undertaken by the Supreme Being. Forms develop over time, however, as a result of processes related to the natural world, such as competition and cooperation between species. The entire universe originates from the Goddess and though changes in life forms will proceed over time, the Goddess remains the lone consciousness permeating all these forms.

Two questions often arise when students are presented with the teaching that a benign, loving Supreme Being created the cosmos. First, if the Goddess is the sole consciousness in existence, from where do destructive forces arise? Second, perhaps a more pointed question, from where arise the evil and selfishness that so pervade humanity?

As regards the first question, when the Goddess offers herself in sacrifice, she emits three primary energies. We might imagine a heavenly fire from which three energies come streaming forth, in the same way that a worldly fire produces smoke, light, and heat. These three energies are the foundation stones of all form and are called *gunas*, literally, "qualities." The three *gunas* are *rajas,* the energy of creation; *tamas,* the energy of destruction; and *sattva,* the energy of balance.

Rajas is in action when forms are generated. When they are being sustained, *sattva* predominates. And when they are destroyed, *tamas* is in effect. The energy that brings seed and egg together in the mother's womb, producing a child and helping it grow, is the energy of *rajas.* The energy which sustains the balance of metabolic and systolic functions necessary for life is that of *sattva.* When the physical form fails to regenerate itself as quickly as it breaks down, old age, and eventually death, result. This is the influence of *tamas.*

The cycle of life is holy in every aspect: the cycle of manifestation/sustenance/and destruction is the holistic expression of the Divine Mother. Destruction is necessary if the life cycle is to continue to revolve. We who admire nature are thrilled to see new growth each spring as fields and forests come alive. But without the occasional lightning storm and resultant fire, the woodland ecosystems would become overgrown with resources too scarce to support the community of plant and animal life. The Mother takes it upon herself to bring about new growth through the destruction of the old.

As for the second question, regarding the origins of evil in humanity, we can say that evil is the result of selfishness, and selfishness arises in individuals who are out of harmony with the Goddess. Though the Goddess is in all people, not all people are aware of her. From the standpoint of Universal Consciousness, no evil can be said to exist, as all is one. In the realm of humanity, however, ignorance and selfishness delay the manifestation of the love and beauty inherent in the Goddess. Selfish forces, therefore, need to be corrected and disciplined. Ethics and morality play an important role in spirituality for human beings. Though ethics may be somewhat relative to cultures, there are certain basic moral principals in yoga— such as non-violence and truthfulness— by which aspirants are expected to abide regardless of circumstances.

5

चितिरेव चेतनपदादवरूढा चेत्यसंकोचिनी चित्तम् ॥

citireva cetanapadādavarūḍhā cetyasaṁkocinī cittam

*It is the Goddess of Universal Consciousness alone
who descends from the realm of infinite awareness.
Becoming limited,
she appears as the subjective beings
and also as the objective phenomenon they perceive.*

This verse is an amplification of the previous verse, again pointing to the one consciousness behind all phenomenon. It is the Goddess herself who becomes the sentient beings in the universe, as well as the various objective, insentient forms which make the props. More precisely, there is a no such thing as insentience, for the entire universe is her mind: space is her mind, rocks are her mind, our bodies are her mind.

All life forms are filled with sentience, regardless of levels of physical or mental activity. The same divine consciousness which animates a human being also permeates a tiger, a tree, and a stone. "Higher" life forms are higher to the extent that they are better able to express the power and freedom of the Goddess, just as a professor of philosophy will be able to articulate the meaning of life better than a toddler. This does not mean the toddler is any less human, or sentient, only that the elder has better developed the tools to express himself.

When one actually perceives all the universe is alive with

consciousness, he/she reaches a very beautiful space, connected with all life. Many people feel themselves alone in the universe, cast adrift in a vast cosmos, isolated within the confines of their bodies and thoughts. The realized soul knows that all individual consciousness is connected in one great consciousness: The Goddess experiences herself through the different aspects of her creation.

In Hindu mythology, this connection is depicted as Indra's Net. Indra is the God of heaven (enlightened perception) and the various strands of his galactic net are woven, with each knot being an individual soul. Each soul is in contact with every other soul via the vibrations it produces. Negative vibrations such as selfishness, anger and fear, are very weak and without the strength to spread very far nor last very long. Positive vibrations, such as compassion, forgiveness and humor, are powerful enough to touch in distant places and have long lasting effects. Love, being one with the Divine Mother, is eternal and omnipresent. As such, whenever love is expressed it touches every soul in the universe and its effect is never-ending. For those who might question this depiction as poetic fancy, the yogi can only respond that this vision is a scientific description of the way energy is transmitted in the universe.

6

तन्मयो मायाप्रमाता ॥

tanmayo māyāpramātā

*The experiencers of this Grand Illusion
are the various individual beings.*

In this verse, we explore the journey of creation through the eyes of the *jiva,* the individual soul. As the *jiva* journeys through the manifest universe, its consciousness evolves through experiences in different life forms. In a human incarnation, the *jiva* has the opportunity to become liberated from identifying with the body/mind complex, and awaken to its true spiritual identity.

I would like to present five stages through which the *jiva* develops along the spiritual path. This is intended to serve as a contextual map which I hope can help aspirants make sense of the major issues they will face in spiritual growth. In writing this, I risk exacerbating a common problem—the tendency of immature aspirants to judge their progress, and that of others, as though they were engaged in some athletic competition in which the goal is to cross the finish line as quickly as possible, and certainly before the other guy.

This competitive attitude, rooted in the ego's desire for separation and status, is blind to two major aspects of the entire spiritual journey. First, spiritual evolution takes place within the Divine Mother's manifestation and, therefore, proceeds at a pace in harmony with Mother herself. This organic process skips no steps, so advancement on the spiritual path is in some ways like physical maturation. It is not better to be 40 years-old than it is 15, though the older person will hopefully be addressing a more subtle set of life issues.

Second, the spiritual journey is entirely comprehensive. The journey begins with the unity of the Goddess and ends with her unity. The separate entity who wishes to advance beyond others is only delaying his own reunion with them. All consciousness is traveling through the cosmos as one. The individual entities are like waves on the same ocean. Large waves have more power than tiny waves, but their "superiority" is only on the surface. Both great and small are part of one magnificent body that ebbs and flows as one.

Stage 1: *Shanti* (Peace)

The first noble truth of the Buddha is *sarvam duhkham,* "all is suffering." Buddhists say this means that the world is like a house on fire, within which we play like little children, unaware of our true situation. The house is our ego, our self-centered, separative identity. Like Midas, with his powerful but horrible touch, our ego-based identity brings suffering to every sphere of life it contacts.

Though this may sound drastic, the realization of the pervasiveness of suffering throughout the manifest universe is an important stage in spiritual growth. Many students initially reject the teachings of the pervasiveness of suffering as overly pessimistic. We think this is how the world must look to somebody in a third-world country surrounded by poverty, starvation, and lack of television. But if we turn the coin around, we can see that our wealth and leisure actually keep us from probing the depth of the human condition. We are so busy with superficialities that we never glimpse below the tip of the iceberg of our small anxieties where mammoth fears and terrors dwell. The pleasures and entertainments that our abundance permit can be seen as activities of endless avoidance.

When we do probe beneath the surface of superficial life we find that, as someone once said, the only thing worse than not getting what you want is getting what you want. All selfish desires are but seeds of discontent. They sprout roots of separative consciousness and branches of competition. They flower in pride and produce the fruit of disappointment, within which are more seeds of discontent. The realization that all ego-based desire results in suffering brings forth the search for its opposite, *shanti,* peace. This longing for peace is the wisdom which begins to untangle the knot of ego.

Stage 2: *Shakti* (Energy)

In the quest for peace, the aspirant comes to the recognition that he/she will need great energy to accomplish all his life tasks without being overwhelmed and stressed-out. The aspirant is drawn to *sadhanas* (spiritual practices) which will improve health as well as stabilize emotions and mental framework. Experiments with diet, sleep, lifestyle, and various formal practices—such as visualization, *pranayama* (breath and energy work) and *asana* (physical postures)—come into play in the pursuit of *shakti.*

During the search for *shakti,* one undergoes processes of purification. To maintain a state of high energy, aspirants realize that the body, emotions, and mind need to be pure and strong, capable of maintaining a high degree of energy. The ordinary person is like a low-wattage light bulb: channel too much electricity through the medium and the bulb will burn out. The aspirants seek to make themselves capable of holding high levels of *shakti,* that they might enjoy the divine luminance.

Purity of body means that the essentials of daily life must be met in a balanced manner. The Ayurvedic medical system, sister science to yoga, states that there are three pillars of life: food, sleep, and sex. Food for an aspirant must be nourishing, fresh, and appropriate to season and lifestyle. A vegetarian diet is extremely helpful for many reasons, though one should not become fanatical about any aspect of diet. After all, it is distraction from the goal itself.

Sleep should be taken in moderation. One should sleep neither too much nor too little. As the body becomes healthy, less sleep is needed because the body is not stressed and wasting the energy it obtained through food, water, air, and sunshine.

Sex, an activity that gives rise to great confusion, is not inherently a barrier to spiritual growth. Sexual activity, within the context of a consensual, mindful relationship, can be an avenue for the maturation of the personality and the satisfaction of the emotions. Sexual behavior, like eating and sleeping, is an issue of exercising moderation and using common sense.

Purity of the emotions and mind means that one learns to remain positive and upbeat. To grow pure, one should look for the noble in all people and God's will in all situations, cultivate attitudes of friendship and compassion towards all other beings, serve as an example of positive energy for those who are dispirited. This is not to imply that life is to be seen through rose-colored glasses. The aspirant should, however, strive to serve as a beacon of happiness in the night of depression and despair in which ego-based persons live. Being happy is amongst the greatest services one can provide for one's brothers and sisters.

Stage 3: *Ramlila* (The Play of God)

As *shakti* develops, the aspirant feels powerful and confident. Life loses its burdensome nature and becomes worthwhile. The insight arises that one's small life is in harmony with the great tides of Mother's creation. And since her nature is joy, likewise does one begin to experience joy in his or her own life.

Spiritual exercises which were previously undertaken in an effort to obtain a goal, such as gaining *shanti* or *shakti*, are now done simply because they are enjoyable. At the early stages of *sadhana*, one feels like a child forced to do homework when play is more inviting. The alarm clock rings in the morning and the beginning yogi wishes for nothing more than to roll over and go back to sleep. S/he does not understand why the teacher requires daily practice. The new yogi would prefer sleep, or coffee and newspaper, to the morning *sadhana*.

Just as the child would rather play games than study, so would the immature yogi favor goofing-off to undertaking practices. Later, however, like a student who has matured and become an enthusiastic scholar, the aspirant looks forward to those periods when s/he can focus on spiritual practices. S/he no longer performs them because something further down the path is sought, but because s/he finds gratification in *sadhana*. Like an artist who enjoys painting, or an athlete who delights in exercise, yogis relishes the opportunity to express their creative life force through *sadhana*.

Stage 4: *Lankabhayankaram* (Terrifier of Lanka)

With the acquisition of the vision of *ramlila,* one might feel that the journey has reached completion. But this is only the prelude to full accomplishment. First, great obstacles which prevent permanent abidance in the sacred inner space must be overcome. From the very depths of the *chitta* (personal consciousness) arise fears, doubts, and defenses which are like a mighty wall obstructing further progress. In psychological terms, we might say that this is the appearance of the darker aspects of the subconscious which are resistant to change. They seek to remain the dominant forces in one's psyche, reluctant to surrender before the tendencies of peace and harmony.

This insight has been presented mythologically in the tales of Christ being tempted in the desert, and of Buddha being attacked by Mara as he sat under the bodhi tree. In both cases the aspirant was victorious. Jesus put Satan behind him and went on to fulfill his mission. The Buddha persisted in his meditation until the forces of Mara were depleted, attaining his supreme enlightenment dedicated to the welfare of all beings.

The term *lankabhayankaram* is an epithet given to Hanuman, one of the heroes of the great Indian epic, the Ramayana, and the focus of part three of this book. *Lankabhayankaram* literally means "terrifier of Lanka," as Hanuman is depicted. He is the destroyer of Lanka, the stronghold of demons. Hanuman is able to recognize a demon, no matter how subtle its disguise, and he holds nothing back in his battle to destroy the negative forces. Symbolically, Hanuman (the accomplished aspirant) is able to recognize the demons (negative thoughts and feelings) which might present themselves to his consciousness, no matter how disguised (attractive, distracting, or logical) they might be. With his mighty club (the power of his own devotion) he destroys their presence in Lanka (in his heart).

Each aspirant must eventually find that fiery part of himself symbolized by Hanuman, the selfless server and noble warrior. The spiritual path is not for the meek or those who give lip service to some amorphous, untested virtue described as "non-violence." Gentleness towards others is always to be demonstrated, but one must be a mighty conqueror of the Lanka within. The demons of selfish desire and laziness will not surrender without a fight. They must be slain with the sword of vitality and enthusiasm for the battle!

Stage 5. *Ma* (Mother)

The primal human sound, Ma, universal throughout virtually every tongue, holds special significance in the yogic tradition. Ma in Sanskrit refers to the Great Goddess, the Divine Mother, the Alpha and Omega of existence. In the final stage of the spiritual journey, the aspirant finds the Goddess laughing in divine intoxication at the blissful paradox of her game of hide and seek.

The Goddess is the peace that surpasses understanding because she lives always beyond the known. She can never be bound by any human concept or limiting idea. In India, she is depicted as Kali, the dancing, black Goddess with a garland of human heads hung on her chest, for all people will be called to offer their heads (egos) to her. They can do so lovingly, in devotion, after which they rise from their beheading reborn as children of God. Or, if ignorance and pride prevent them from humbly submitting themselves to this process, Kali ends up with their heads anyway through the defeats that life heaves upon the egoic person, ending with the supreme defeat, the humiliation of death.

Yoga is a rational system of steps that lead to this fifth stage, the transrational leap of faith into that which can never be known, only loved. Depicting this transcendence as Goddess is very appropriate for our time, for we have become estranged from nature and the feminine values of sympathy, tenderness, and an appreciation for the cyclical nature of life.

Our rocket ships, our computers, and our atom bombs prove our ability to construct devices that demonstrate our cleverness at applying reason and manipulating Aristotelian logic. Great as these achievements might be, they leave us empty in heart, for the heart is the realm of intuition. Like Adam and Eve, we have tasted the fruits of our knowing, only to find how bitter is the cost.

I am not proposing that we abandon reason, only that it be informed by intuition. For unless we are able, when necessary, to leap from the rational mind into the intuitive heart, our earthly accomplishments are nothing but dust. And, as our weapons of destruction suggest, we may end as dust if we don't heed the voice of this inner Goddess.

Bedecked with her garland of severed heads, she appears dark and frightening only because she lives in the shadows of our unconscious. As one progresses through the stages of spiritual growth, one comes to know that fear of her is nothing more than a self-perpetuating illusion based on ignorance.

Aspirant, fear nothing! Doubt your doubts, be angry with your anger, and penetrate through the darkness of terror-induced nightmares to the bliss soaked dance of divine life: born, sustained, and then destroyed by Ma.

Of Kali, Swami Vivekananda wrote:

> Dancing mad with joy,
> Come, Mother. Come!
> For terror is Thy name,
> Death is in Thy breath,
> And every shaking step
> destroys a world for e'er.
> Thou 'Time', the All-Destroyer!
> Come, O' Mother. Come!
> Who dares misery love,
> And hug the form of Death,
> Dance in destruction's dance,
> To him the Mother comes. *

7

स चैको द्विरूपस्त्रिमयश्चतुरात्मा सप्तपञ्चकस्वभावः ॥

sa caiko dvirūpastrimayaścaturātmā saptapañcakasvabhāvaḥ

Although God's essential nature is unitary,
she manifests as duality, as three-fold nature,
as the fourfold soul, and as seven pentads.

This verse describes the cosmology and ontology of the tantric system. Other ontologies exist in Indian spiritual traditions, amongst which the Samkhya system which Patanjali employed is the most well known. The system presented here is the most complete, however, identifying every aspect of our universe, from the most cosmic to the sub-atomic. It is worth recognizing the depth of insight the ancient seers had into the realms of both spirit and the material world. This text was written some 1000 years ago, yet it anticipates modern discoveries in sub-atomic and quantum physics, giving credence to the claims of the great yogis that human beings can develop powers of perception for which modern man has needed tools such as telescopes and microscopes.

* Nivedita, Sister, [M.E. Noble]*Kali the Mother (*Advaita Ashrama, Majavati, Almora) 1953.

The unitary nature of God is the highest realm of consciousness. All aspects of divinity originate from this level. Here, God and Goddess, complete transcendence and complete eminence, are one. At this level the dialectic opposites existing in every realm of existence are resolved in one absolute containing all. This consciousness is beyond the reach of the mind; silence is the only language that can express its reality.

The dual nature of God was first discussed in the preface and is covered in various parts of this work. Worth mentioning here, however, are the multitude of metaphors used in the different yogic traditions to symbolize this dual nature. The Shaivites refer to Shiva and Shakti; the Vaishnavas to Krishna and Radha, or Rama and Sita; the *raja* yogis to Purusha and Prakriti; and Hindus throughout India recognize Vishnu and Lakshmi, and Brahma and Saraswati. The essential teaching held in common throughout these different traditions is that the one God is, in essence, of a two-fold nature: eternally transcendent, while at the same time eternally immanent.

The three-fold nature of God here refers to the three *gunas,* or qualities of nature. As discussed in verse 4, the three *gunas* function under the direction of the Great Mother in creating, sustaining, and destroying all forms. Besides the macrocosmic realms of creation, the *gunas* also operate on the microcosmic realms.

In human experience, the three *gunas* influence an individual's physical, emotional, and mental make-up. The *gunas* are the determining factor in the level of consciousness of individual human beings. As one aligns oneself with *tamas*, consciousness will be lethargic and self-centered. As one aligns with *rajasic* energies, one becomes overactive and seeks others who agree with his or her values while condemning those who disagree. The one who aligns with *sattva* becomes peaceful and sees all people as brothers and sisters.

How the three *gunas* operate within the psyche is expressed in the following parable. A man is walking along a path when he is attacked by three robbers. They bind him and take his money. Then they debate his fate. The first robber says, "He is no good to us anymore. Let's kill him and bury his body in a ditch."

The second robber argues that death is too harsh, but he is worried that the man will turn them in if he is found alive. He proposes, "Let us blindfold him, and put him deep into the forest. If he is eaten by wild animals it would not be our fault."

The third robber tells the other two that he will take care of the problem of dealing with their victim and they can go ahead with their escape. The third robber then unbinds the man and helps dress his wounds. He gives the man food and water and volunteers to walk him to his village so he won't be attacked by other bandits.

As the two reach the outskirts of the village, the robber, in a feeling of remorse, returns to the man his portion of the stolen money. The man is so touched that he invites the robber to come to his home and stay with his family as a guest. The robber declines the invitation, however, because his reputation as a thief is well known and he is certain to be apprehended by the police if he enters the town.

The first robber represents *tamas guna*. All he wanted was to take care of his own desires. After that, as far as he was concerned, the man could be eliminated. *Tamas guna* makes an individual entirely self-centered, without concern for the well-being of others.

The second robber represents *rajas guna*. He got what he wanted, so he was willing to show some mercy on the man. *Rajas guna* makes an individual selfish, but still willing to help others as long as it doesn't interfere with his own happiness.

The third robber represents *sattva guna*. It makes one compassionate and able to see his own mistakes. *Sattva guna* inspires a person to strive to do what is right and make amends for what is wrong. But *sattva guna* is still unable to enter the town, symbolizing divine consciousness. *Sattva guna* is still a "thief," a limiting condition, and is therefore only able to exist outside the boundaries of divine consciousness. *Sattva guna* is the energy of nature which enables an aspirant to reach the gate of higher consciousness, but it cannot accompany the aspirant there. The soul must leave behind all the *gunas* to reach home in higher consciousness.

The soul is identified as being fourfold because the psychic apparatus of an individual, called the *antahkarana*, consists of four aspects: *manas, buddhi, ahamkara,* and *chitta. Manas* is the aspect of mind which collates and organizes the information that the senses receive from their interaction with the external world.

Buddhi is the intellect, which identifies and classifies the picture of reality that *manas* constructs. *Ahamkara* is the individual identity, the ego, which claims ownership of the mental and sensory phenomenon and judges it's value as essentially pleasurable or painful. *Chitta* is the substratum of consciousness, which records experiences and holds the sum and substance of the experiences in the forms of seeds of desires and motivations called *samskaras.* The functions of the *antahkarana* will be amplified in verse 1 of the *Nirvanashatkam.*

The seven pentads refer to the way in which the five energies of Shiva (to be discussed in verse 11) manifest through the seven *chakras* within a human being. In tantric traditions it is said that the spiritual journey is about 36 inches long, from the base of the spine to the crown of the skull. This refers to the distance the *kundalini* must travel from the lowest to the highest *chakra*, from the alpha point to the omega point.

Kundalini is the energy of the great Goddess within the human form, supplying consciousness and energy. After the human body is built by material energies, *kundalini* descends through the crown of the head and rests at the base of the spine. Here she lays as potential, untapped by the majority of humanity, for genius, for inspired creativity, and for spiritual accomplishment.

Yogis attempt to engage in a relationship with *kundalini* and precipitate her rise up the *chakras*.

The *chakras* abide in the *sushumna*, which is said to lay "inside" the spinal cord. It should be made clear, however, that there exist no *chakras*, no *sushumna*, and no *kundalini* on the physical plane. No *chakras* have ever been found upon autopsy of a human body. These energies lay in the subtle body, where they are as real as flesh and blood for the physical body. During the course of their spiritual practices, yogis experience first-hand the reality of the *chakras* and of the *kundalini*.

The following chart designates the nature of the *chakra* system, reviewing some of the principals introduced in verse 3.

Chakra	Location	Influence
Sahasrara	crown of head	union with God
Ajna	forehead	spiritual insight
Vishuddha	behind throat	inspired creativity
Anahata	behind sternum	compassion
Manipura	behind solar plexus	individual vitality
Svadhisthana	behind genitals	sensuality
Muladhara	base of spine	attachment to body

8

तद्भूमिकाः सर्वदर्शनस्थितयः ॥

tadbhūmikāḥ sarvadarśanasthitayaḥ

All systems of philosophy are limited viewpoints
from which only a portion
of the unitary whole
is seen and described.

This verse is expressive of the pervasive idea in Indian philosophy that "Truth is one, the wise call it by many names." This understanding provides the key for the resolution of all philosophical debates and for the eradication of dogmatic fundamentalism. All systems of philosophy are somewhat true and somewhat false. Each is accurate, but limited, because it presents just one of an infinite number of perspectives and level of consciousness. Every philosophy depicts the universe from a vantage point which is true to the extent that it represents the vision of the

Goddess, and false to the extent that it is influenced by the ego. No philosopher can claim to understand all the workings of God. That privilege belongs only to the Divine Mother.

It might be said that the entire purpose of manifestation is to give the Goddess an opportunity to reflect upon herself and contemplate her own nature. Philosophy is the human endeavor of attempting to understand and appreciate the activity of the eternal Mother. It is her delight and pleasure to incarnate as human beings who attempt to fathom her. This *Pratyabhijna Hridayam* is part of her play, a love letter to herself across time and space, detailing how she originated the universe and how we, as manifestations of her, can enjoy the experience of being human.

Over the past few centuries, philosophic study and academic research has been on the wane in the yogic tradition as a whole. In large part, this has been a healthy revolt against the over-intellectualized approach of the brahminic heritage. For in authentic yogic traditions, philosophy is never intended to be an armchair sport. Scholars are expected to also be practitioners of spiritual disciplines.

9

चिद्वत्तच्छक्तिसंकोचात् मलावृतः संसारी ॥

cidvattacchaktisaṁkocāt malāvṛtaḥ saṁsārī

The self-limitation of Universal Energy
results in the Goddess of Universal Consciousness
becoming transformed into personal beings
enmeshed in divine forgetfulness.

This verse presents a more detailed analysis of the nature of the transformation of Universal Consciousness into individuated personal beings. In the tantra tradition, this transformation is described as the result of the binding of the five-fold *kancuka,* "coverings." In his *Yoga Sutras,* Patanjali also designated bondage as being five-fold in his brilliant exegesis on the *kleshas,* "afflictions."

Let us compare both systems in hope of shedding some light on this crucial spiritual issue:

Level	Tantra	Raja Yoga	Bondage
1.	Kalaa	Avidya	"I am an individual."
2.	Vidya	Asmita	"I am an individual body & mind."
3.	Raga	Raga	"I am an individual body & mind with desires to fulfill."
4.	Kaala	Dvesha	"I am an individual, temporal body and mind with desires to fulfill and dislikes to avoid."
5.	Niyati	Abhinivesha	"I am an individual, temporal body and mind with desires to fulfill and dislikes to avoid, and one day I shall, unfortunately, die."

In each of the five levels, there is a progressive reduction in Universal Consciousness and a deepening of identification with a body/mind complex. The first level of bondage is called *kalaa* in tantra, and *avidya* by the raja yogis. It is the level at which Universal Consciousness is wrapped in a cocoon of ignorance and awareness of her true nature is hidden. At this level, individuality arises separate from the universal, along with an intrinsic desire to sustain that individuality. At this level arises the feeling, "I am an individual."

The second level of bondage is called *vidya,* and *asmita*. Here the omniscience of the Universal Consciousness is reduced to the sentience of an individual being limited by the instruments of cognition. At this level arises the feeling, "I am an individual body and mind."

The third level of bondage is called *raga* in both traditions. Here the complete satisfaction of the Universal Consciousness is reduced, bringing about a desire for objects perceived outside of the individual body. At this level arises the feeling, "I am an individual body and mind with desires to fulfill."

The fourth level of bondage is called *kaala*, and *dvesha*. This is the companion to the bondage of the third level and the other side of the coin of desire. Here arises the impulse to avoid objects which seem to hamper satisfaction. At this level arises the feeling, "I am an individual, temporal body and mind with desires to fulfill and dislikes to avoid."

The fifth level of bondage is called *niyati*, and *abhinivesha*. Here the Omnipresence of the Universal Consciousness is reduced, producing an attachment to the individual body/mind complex and a corresponding fear of death. At this level arises the feeling, "I am an individual, temporal body and mind with desires to fulfill and dislikes to avoid, and one day I shall, unfortunately, die."

We can see how these five *kancukas/kleshas* grow from an initial ignorance of spiritual reality into identity with a body/mind complex. This identification is reinforced with likes and dislikes, and results in attachment to form and fear of death. In Patanjali's school, as well as in many Vedantic traditions, these bonds are seen as basically evils to be overcome for the soul to attain its freedom. In this *Pratyabhijna Hridayam,* as in other tantric and devotional schools, the bonds are seen in the light of the *lila*, the playful spirit of God. The Goddess wraps herself in these cloaks by her own device, for the sheer joy of later unraveling them through love and devotion. Like a caterpillar who enters a cocoon, later to emerge as a beautiful butterfly, the Divine Mother enters the world in the form of the individual souls in order to express her own vitality and beauty.

10

तथापि तद्वत् पञ्चकृत्यानि करोति ॥

tathāpi tadvat pañcakṛtyāni karoti

Even while in the condition of the limited personal being,
the Universal Consciousness
still performs the five great acts.

Indian philosophy is frequently denigrated by westerners as being world-negative. There is some truth to the charge, but the world-negating position is actually just one part of Indian spirituality. The tantric tradition, which the *Pratyabhijna Hridayam* presents, has always been world positive. The world, with all of its changes and forms, is none other than the divine Goddess herself. The tantrist does not seek to transcend the world; s/he seeks to transcend personal illusion so s/he might be in harmony with the world and see it in its true, glorious light.

The five-fold act referred to in this verse is performed on a universal scale by the Goddess, and on a personal level by the individual human being. The five acts are described in detail in the next verse, so we will not examine them too closely here. The point being made in this verse is that the nature of the Goddess is being expressed at all times, in all forms.

The Goddess descends into the realm of human consciousness, but even at this level she continues to play her divine game. To those who can feel her reality, life's events are all part of a "carnival of joy," as the great Kali worshipper, Paramahansa Ramakrishna put it. This idea can be understood by the intellect, but intellectual understanding is not sufficient to bring about the change in consciousness necessary to actually perceive this reality: to see the Goddess and to dance with her.

Intellectual understanding is like looking at a picture of fire. Only the reality of fire is sufficient to cook food or warm one's home on a cold evening. Placing a picture of a fire underneath one's cook pot will not provide nourishment. To enter into the unity of the Goddess, one must be willing to transcend the intellect with a leap of intuition.

I would like here to issue a word of caution to aspirants. To transcend the intellect does not mean that one becomes irrational. Rather, the rational mind remains as an efficient tool for dealing with activities of life requiring linear thought. But it is not in the intellect that the Goddess will be found.

The intellect makes a fine office, but the holy shrine is found in the intuitive heart.

11

आभासन-रक्ति-विमर्शन-बीजावस्थापन-विलापनतस्तानि ॥

ābhāsana-rakti-vimarśana-bījāvasthāpana-vilāpanatastāni

These five great acts are:
manifesting, enjoying, identification,
proliferation, and dissolution.

The five "great acts," or functions of the Universal Consciousness are the five movements in the Divine Mother's dance. The first is manifesting, or creating. The primal creative spark arises from the infinitely energetic impulse of the Goddess. This spark is not the immediate cause of everything that exists, but it is the initial impulse behind all manifestation and all individual creative ideas and actions. We would not, for instance, say the Goddess created the Brooklyn Bridge, but we could say she created humanity's ability to inspire itself with such a grand idea. The creative activity of the Goddess is inherently enjoyable to her. Enjoyment, therefore, is the second function of the Universal Consciousness.

The Goddess acts out the third function of identification by fully entering into her creation. She loses herself, in a sense, by identifying completely with her creations. In wild, care-free abandon she allows her identity to become absorbed into the limited forms and consciousness of individual beings.

The fourth function of the Goddess is proliferation. We see this in the immense abundance of nature. A single blade of wild grass holds thousands of seeds, all capable of themselves becoming plants bearing thousands, maybe millions of additional seeds. The bounty of nature is so overwhelming that it beguiles the mind. When we come into harmony with this abundance, our lives become rich with the bounty that is our inheritance as children of the eternally creative Divine Mother.

The fifth function of the Goddess is dissolution. Here she commands the forces of destruction and transformation. This model of

Divinity provides for the resolution of personal fears and anxieties about death. For death is not the enemy of life, it is simply a transformation. Death is only the dissolution of form. The essence of life is eternal: it was never born and it can never die. The Divine Mother holds her children in her arms during their birth, during their lives, and during their deaths.

12

तदपरिज्ञाने स्वशक्तिभिर्व्यामोहितता संसारित्वम ॥

tadaparijñāne svaśaktibhirvyāmohitatā saṁsāritvam

A personal being is one who
is enchanted by a sense of possessing power,
and lacks the wisdom to discern
that the Goddess of Universal Consciousness
is actually the performer of the five great acts.

This is a further amplification of the principal identified initially in verse 4, that the individual being is really the Goddess herself in disguise. In previous verses this was discussed from the macrocosmic standpoint of the Goddess cloaking herself in the various levels of consciousness and grades of matter. Here the limitation of Universal Consciousness is approached from a more microcosmic, psychological orientation, reflecting the way individual human beings perceive themselves.

The great devotee of Kali, Ram Prasad, sings:

> Everything is your desire, Supreme Desire, O' Dear Mother.
> All actions you perform, Ma, still people say that I have done.
> I am a tool, you are the craftsman,
> I am a house, you are the master.
> I am a car, you are the driver.
> Just as you drive, just so I run. *

---

* From *The Songs of Ramprasad* by Shree Maa, copyright 1996 by Devi Mandir.

From the standpoint of the Absolute reality, there are no individual beings. From the relative plane where differences are manifest, individuality most certainly exists. If I eat, you may still go hungry. But to the enlightened devotee like Ram Prasad, his own consciousness is nothing more than a wave on the infinite ocean of the Goddess. Waves rise and fall, exist and subside, but the ocean itself is forever.

If the Goddess is the sole performer of actions, does the limited individual actually have any free-will? The answer is "Yes, but only to an extent." The Goddess alone has complete free-will, all other beings are limited in their potency and freedom. Like a horse within a fenced field, the individual has free-will up to a certain point. He can run around within the field that his *karma* allows, but beyond that he cannot pass. Only by transcending his limited identity can he pass beyond the boundaries that *karma* imposes and enjoy the freedom of enlightenment.

13

तत्परिज्ञाने चित्तमेव अन्तर्मुखीभावेन चेतनपदाध्यारोहात् चितिः ॥

tatparijñāne cittameva antarmukhībhāvena cetanapadādhyārohāt citiḥ

Upon intuiting that the Goddess of Universal Consciousness
is the sole performer of the five great acts,
the individual consciousness of the aspirant
is developed by directing it internally in meditation.
The aspirant ascends to the realm of pure consciousness
and realizes identity with her.

This verse deals with the *upaya*, or meditative technique, describing more precisely how the aspirant is to transcend the sense of limited individuality and realize identity with the Goddess. The aspirant has glimpsed the reality of the Goddess and his/her relationship to her, but s/he is not stabilized in that elevated stage of consciousness. Hence the aspirant must perform spiritual practices such as meditation. In this verse there are four stages described in the development of the aspirant's consciousness:

1. One intuits the Goddess is the performer of the five acts.
2. One begins to develop one's consciousness through meditation.
3. One ascends to the realm of pure consciousness.
4. One realizes one's identity with the Goddess.

In the first stage, the aspirant attains the intuitive insight that it is the Goddess who is actually the performer of the five functions. One's personal mind and body are, as Ram Prasad wrote, her vehicle, her tool, her instrument. The individual is the altar upon which the flame of the Goddess rests. The altar is to be honored for the role it plays in the grand scheme of life, but it is the living flame, not the altar, which is to be worshipped.

In the second stage, the aspirant deliberately undertakes meditative disciplines for the purpose of cultivating spiritual consciousness. Specific *sadhanas* will be practiced everyday based on advice given by a *guru* or on intuitive understanding. The main principal of meditative practices is the internalization of consciousness. The aspirant dives into his or her own being in an effort to pierce the veils of physical, emotional and mental life in order to find the true spiritual self. In addition to internal practices, daily life comes to revolve around one's spiritual goal, so activities of daily life are performed in a manner which is efficient and enhances spiritual growth. When internal disciplines and external life come into harmony, the aspirant has attained to a high level and will make increasingly swift progress.

In the third stage, the aspirant has accomplished the goal of *sadhana*. S/he has become cleansed of selfishness and fear, and consciousness is enlightened. Like a pond that has had algae cleared from its surface, the aspirant's consciousness is now resplendent and life giving. The mind and heart radiate wisdom and compassion. The aspirant becomes a saint.

The fourth stage is one which is beyond accomplishment, since it occurs by the will of the Goddess. An aspirant may climb to the summit of pure consciousness (the third stage) but here s/he will have to wait patiently for the Goddess' embrace in her own sweet time. But when this embrace occurs, the soul of the aspirant merges into the Goddess like a raindrop entering the sea. Actually, the experience is more like the sea entering the raindrop. For the Goddess's evolutionary game is enhanced by the savoring of all individual experiences within the immensity of her cosmic consciousness. Nothing undergone by the individual consciousness is lost; rather, it finds its proper place in the Mother's heart. Just as every living creature has a unique niche in the earth's ecosystem, a niche which is essential for the entire web of life to function, likewise, each individual experience is a necessary cell in the cosmic body of the Mother.

14

चितिवह्निरवरोहपदे छन्नोऽपि मात्रया मेयेन्धनं प्लुष्यति ॥

citivahniravarohapade channo'pi mātrayā meyendhanaṁ pluṣyati

As the Goddess descends to lower realms of consciousness
where her universality is concealed,
external objects serve as various grades of fuel
for the fire of her Universal Consciousness.

The descent of the Goddess is undertaken for her own pleasure and amusement. As she descends into the lower realms, the unification of her pure consciousness is fragmented in the same way that white light is fragmented through a prism. When the Goddess descends, her pure sound, the primal *Aum* vibration, is broken into an unlimited number of separate songs. The various individual beings throughout time and space sing their own unique songs, each of which is a single note in the universal choir of the eternal *Aum*. The descent of the Goddess creates the different forms, which are the instruments through which is played the song of life.

Objects serve as the stimuli, or fuel, for the experiences of individual beings. The consciousness of an individual is like a fire of a certain degree of potency and purity. This fire is capable of responding to, or "burning," only a certain portion of the cosmos within its flames. This portion of the universe that is burned is the realm of experience that the individual knows as his personal universe. The greater the fire of consciousness, the more of the universe the individual will be capable of experiencing and understanding.

For millennia, yogis in India have performed ceremonies involving building a sacred fire, and making offerings into it of *mantras,* songs, and prayers. These ceremonies are an external, exoteric reflection of an internal, esoteric process. The inner ceremony involves building a strong fire of consciousness and offering into it the experiences of life. For the enlightened sage, the entire universe is a beautiful ceremonial offering of love, song, and joy.

15

बललाभे विश्वमात्मसात्करोति ॥

balalābhe viśvamātmasātkaroti

On attaining mastery,
the individual soul
embodies the universe.

In many schools of Indian mysticism, it is believed that the union of the individual soul with God can occur only after death. Other schools, including the Pratyabhijna school, hold that an individual may attain the state of *jiva-mukti,* liberated while still incarnated.

The schools that argue death is necessary fail to understand an essential principal of the revelatory union of the individual and the supreme. They hold that an individual being cannot experience totality because the ego must first be relinquished. Since the ego is the unifying principal around which body and mind function, they reason that without an ego there would be no centralized energy to continue to coordinated life processes. They fail to realize, however, that the ego need not be destroyed for totality to be experienced, it must only be transcended. The ego can remain to help coordinate functions of body and mind without interfering with the union of consciousness.

"I am a . . . man, woman, Christian, Hindu, etc." The *jiva-mukti,* however, sees clearly that egoic identity is nothing more than a combination of bodily identification and social conditioning. In deep meditation the *jiva-mukti* dissolves this false identity and experiences the self as one with the Goddess of Universal Consciousness. S/he then joins with the Goddess in experiencing the entire universe as her body.

In order to continue to participate in the worlds of manifestation, the sage may deliberately adopt a provisional ego. Unlike the ego of the ordinary person, however, the ego of the accomplished yogi is consciously created. It is not the result of external programming, but of deliberate, willful consideration. The ego created by the *jiva-mukti* proclaims, "I am a devotee." The devotee/*jiva-mukti* is able to experience the bliss of union with the Goddess, as well as the joy of participating in the cosmic drama as her worshipper.

16

चिदानन्दलाभे देहादिषु चेत्यमानेष्वपि
चिदैकात्म्यप्रतिपत्तिदाढर्यं जीवन्मुक्तिः ॥

cidānandalābhe dehādiṣu cetyamāneṣvapi
cidaikātmyapratipattidārḍhyaṁ jīvanmuktiḥ

The evolving soul who has attained
the bliss of the Goddess of Universal Consciousness,
and is firmly established in the awareness that
all processes of the body/mind network
are objective phenomenon,
is deemed liberated while still in incarnation.

This verse enhances our understanding of the *jiva-mukti,* the one who is liberated while still in incarnation. The enlightened soul experiences the self as pure subjectivity, separate from the body/mind complex. The body and mind are like the cart and horse the soul rides during incarnation.

For many people, the horse of their mind runs on its own volition and does not obey the orders of its master. It gallops here and there, hungry one minute, tired the next, and wild and unruly after that. The soul which is not in control of the mind cannot accomplish any spiritual work in this world. In fact, myriad incarnations are spent as a soul learns to operate the "machinery" of body and mind. As the evolving soul becomes more accomplished at this task, s/he is able to spend less time during incarnation learning how to control the vehicles, and more time using them for spiritual growth and service to others.

This verse highlights the ideal of the *jiva-mukti.* As discussed in the commentary to the previous verse, many schools of Indian philosophy, including most of Buddhism, and many of the Vedanta schools, believe that liberation is only possible after the death of the body. The body, incarnation, even the entire physical universe, are seen as painful experiences which are to be escaped from as quickly as possible. This very pervasive notion is reminiscent of the Christian Gnostic teachings which believe in a brilliant soul trapped in the mud of the physical body.

The *Pratyabhijna Hridayam* presents a different view of incarnation, one which honors the manifest world and the various forms which comprise physical existence. The world is seen as an emanation of the Goddess, the very body of the Goddess. It is to be honored and treated with the utmost respect. Incarnation in a physical form is not seen as a punishment or the result of bad karma, but for the purpose of celebrating the abundance of love abiding in the heart of the Goddess.

To achieve "liberation," one does not need to escape from the "prison" of the body. One need only escape from the erroneous identification of the soul with the body/mind complex. When the body is recognized as being a temporary vehicle for the soul, it finds its rightful place in the grand harmony of creation. The body is respected without being worshipped, and treated properly without being adored. The soul experiences itself as separate from the body, but does not disdain the vehicle which makes service in this world possible.

The *Pratyabhijna* philosophy provides a context in which the body and all of nature are seen in love, harmony, and beauty. Relationships and family life, sexuality, art, music, and recreation all have the potential to serve as appropriate vehicles for the creative energy underlying the universe. Physical and social life need not burden the soul; they can be extensions of the soul's consuming desire to express love for the creator.

17

मध्यविकासाच्चिदानन्दलाभः ॥

madhyavikāsāccidānandalābhāḥ

As the center of consciousness blossoms,
the individual soul attains
the bliss of the Goddess of Universal Consciousness.

This verse is a further amplification of the appreciation for the creative expression mentioned in verse 16. In many traditions, the aspirant is asked to withdraw consciousness from all contact with the external world in order to find freedom. Though meditative inversion is not antithetical to this text, the *Pratyabhijna* philosophy proposes that consciousness does not develop by escaping from anything. Rather, consciousness develops by exhibiting its potential and fulfilling its great purpose.

Consciousness expands in the same way that a flower grows: from the center out. This center, the *hridayam* of the title of this text, is an eternal fount of love. To stifle its expression through negativity and

disdain for manifested life is opposed to the vision of life being presented. For the flower of consciousness to grow, it must live in the soil of
gratitude for the gift of incarnation.

To seek to remove oneself from incarnate experience is to deny
the *shakti* of the Goddess. The playful purpose of the Goddess is to plant
herself like a field of flowers, so the splendor of her beauty can shine in
greater and greater expanses.

18

विकल्पक्षय शक्तिसंकोचविकास वाहच्छेदाद्न्तकोटि
निभालनादय इहोपायाः ॥

vikalpakṣaya śaktisaṁkocavikāsa vāhacchedādyantakoṭi
nibhālanādaya ihopāyaḥ

The skillful means to develop this center include:
quieting the modifications which
form individual perception;
becoming aware of the manner
by which consciousness exteriorizes and is withdrawn;
controlling the two fundamental life energies;
and seeing into the cycle of existence.

The science of yoga, like any science, is based on a foundation of
logic and replicabilty. Sri Swami Rama of the Himalayas said, "Yoga is a
divine science that furnishes the means to educate and develop the whole
person." Georg Feuerstein has correctly identified yoga as a "technology
of ecstasy," and Paramahansa Yogananda said yoga is as precise as
mathematics. Yoga is definitely a verb: it is a series of practices which are
undertaken by an aspirant intent on realizing the true nature of oneself
and the world. This verse presents the manner of these practices from the
Pratyabhijna standpoint.

The first practice recommended in this verse is quieting the modifications which form individual perception. These modifications, or *vikalpas,* are the habitual tendencies of the mind to reinforce its own limited identity. When the *vikalpas* begin to subside, the aspirant perceives how his personal identity is largely based on sensory interactions, mental formations, and psychological projections. To transcend personal identity and realize spiritual identity, the *vikalpas* must be quieted through regular spiritual practice.

The second practice mentions the ability to interiorize consciousness. In a number of Eastern traditions, this ability is given the utmost significance. The goal of these traditions is to attain *samadhi,* deep meditative trance. Reaching *samadhi* is no small achievement, as it provides the meditator with the direct experience of the self as separate from the body/mind complex. But the ability to interiorize consciousness is only half the goal presented by the *Pratyabhijna Hridayam.*

This text describes the goal of spiritual practice as the ability to control the flow of awareness in both of its movements—internally and externally. When consciousness can be deeply internalized, the aspirant attains *nirvikalpa samadhi,* "absorption in the transcendent." When the yogi is able to control the externalization of consciousness through his or her body, mind, and senses, s/he attains *bhava samadhi,* "absorption in divine emotions," and realizes the Goddess, eternal movement. These two *samadhis* are expressive of the dual nature of divinity.

The cycle of existence—interiorization and exteriorization—is the great cycle of cosmic life. The two components of the cycle are known in yogic philosophy as *pravritti,* or manifestation, and *nivritti,* or interiorization.

The Goddess engages in *pravritti* during the periods of her creation of the universe, and she engages in *nivritti* during the re-absorption of the universe back into herself at the end of a cycle. The accomplished yogi comes into harmony with this cycle as s/he goes deeply within in *nirvikalpa samadhi,* and extends consciousness outward in *bhava samadhi.*

19

समाधिसंस्कारवति व्युत्थाने भूयो
भूयश्चिदैक्यामर्शान्नित्योदितसमाधिलाभः ॥

samādhisaṁskāravati vyutthāne bhūyo
bhūyaścidaikyāmarśānnityoditasamādhilābhaḥ

After the initial experiences of samadhi,
one will return to customary consciousness
but will carry impressions of the experience.
To permanently abide in union
with the Goddess of Universal Consciousness,
one will need to repeatedly practice samadhi.

When a yogi first experiences the beauty and profundity of *samadhi* during spiritual practice, s/he inevitably believes that the goal has been achieved and s/he has attained abiding union with the Goddess. This mistake is due to a mis-perception by the yogi of the timelessness experienced in *samadhi*. S/he finds time transcended in *samadhi,* but the yogi will return to the subjective experience of linear time when s/he comes back to ordinary consciousness.

The descent from *samadhi* can be confusing. In this elevated state the yogi knows the self to be one with all the universe, while s/he later identifies again with an individual body/mind complex. The benefits of *samadhi* include the knowledge that individual identity is a temporary phenomenon. The *vikalpas* of personal perception and identity are reduced, and the *kleshas* that cover the soul's brilliant light are shredded.

The descent from *samadhi* reveals to the honest yogi those aspects of consciousness which limit the ability to access *samadhi* at will. Mother Nature insists that one who wishes to abide in her innermost chambers is free of selfishness, anger, greed, fear, and attachment. After the experience of *samadhi,* the return to human consciousness will be disturbing. But the "taste" of *samadhi* remains in the mind, acting as a polestar by which the aspiring yogi can direct life's journey.

20

तदा प्रकाशानन्दसारमहामन्त्रवीर्यात्मकपूर्णाहंतावेशात् सदा
सर्वसर्गसंहारकारि निजसंविद्देवताचक्रेश्वरताप्राप्तिर्भवतीति शिवम् ॥

tadā prakāśānandasāramahāmantravīryātmakapūrṇāhaṁtāveśāt
sadā sarvasargasaṁhārakāri
nijasaṁviddevatācakreśvaratāprāptirbhavatīti śivam

With repeated practice of samadhi,
personal consciousness reaches it's completion,
and the soul realizes its essence as bliss and light.
The soul comes to know the power within its own being
as the great mantra,
and the everlasting cycle of creation and re-absorption.
Personal consciousness is transcended,
and the soul realizes mastery over all the deities
in its sphere of consciousness.
The individual soul has become the expression
of the infinite kindness and compassion
of the Divine Mother.

With repeated immersion in *samadhi,* the individualized consciousness becomes Divine Consciousness. The evolutionary journey reaches its peak in an alchemical transformation as the once bound soul becomes one with bliss and light. The soul is no longer a mere reflection of the Goddess; it becomes an active agent of her will, resounding the great *mantra* of Being throughout the cosmos.

Like all yogic cosmologies, the *Pratyabhijna Hridayam* acknowledges the existence of consciousness and life-forms superior to those we know on the human realm. These higher beings are superior to humanity in terms of their life-span, power, and the degrees of wisdom and bliss they experience. Nonetheless, all beings are emanations of the Mother and, from that perspective, are equal. Mother loves all her children to the maximum level. The highly evolved are simply more aware of this divine love, and are able to serve as conscious conduits for her in the manifest worlds. The soul who realizes its true identity in the Divine Mother is enlightened to to a state of primal supremacy and mastery over all.

The enlightened one realizes all exists within one's being. Swami Rama Tirtha said, "I am in all, and all is in me." He had become immersed in the Divine Mother and her all-encompassing love, her infinite kindness and compassion. In the form of the enlightened soul, the Goddess of Universal Consciousness fully manifests her glory in the world.

Conclusion

The sanskrit original of the *Pratyabhijna Hridayam* closes with a brief statement by Kshemaraja. He offers the text to those who sincerely seek the truth of life, but do not have the scholarly skills required for the full study of the *Pratyabhijna* philosophy. He therefore offers this synopsis, the essence of the matter: the heart of Self-Realization. He acknowledges his appreciation for his most venerable *guru,* Abhinavagupta, and he brings his work to a close with these words:

"May all enjoy
the infinite kindness and compassion
of the Goddess of Universal Consciousness."

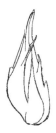

Part II

The Transcendent God

In this section we will explore the *Nirvanashatkam,* "Six Verses on Nirvana," a concise presentation of *jnana* yoga, the yoga of wisdom. Shankara, the author, is one of India's most revered saints. His life of only 33 years took place sometime around 700 AD. During this time he wrote commentaries on many of the most important scriptures, and traveled the length and breadth of India preaching and establishing monastic centers. Several of the lineages he established are still vital today.

Shankara taught that the goal of spirituality is the realization of the eternal, formless, absolute, transcendent Godhead. He believed that theism and deity worship were lower forms of spirituality. He argued that creation is an illusory phenomenon, and the notion of a personal God is just an idea held in the minds of unenlightened men. Shankara's teachings exalt the gnostic focus of the *Upanishads* that an individual must find the truth within.

The *Nirvanashatkam* is a remarkable, if somewhat difficult, text. It depicts a radical *advaita,* non-dualism. This non-dualism is based on the premise that one's true identity is transcendent to the body/mind complex. One's real identity is the conscious Self, which is the pure sense of "I am." When the "I am" consciousness identifies with a body, delusion arises in the form of the thought, "I am an individual, independent body and mind." Liberation, from this perspective, is the detachment of the pure consciousness of "I am" from deluded identification with the body and mind.

Advaita is described as the narrow spiritual path without handrails. It demands a fierce detachment and intellectual austerity that can be daunting. All temporal phenomenon, including the idea of personal deity, must be sacrificed if one is to reach the Absolute. In the context of the *Nirvanashatkam,* Shankara refers to the Absolute as "Shiva."

In this text we are attending to the completely transcendent. The Shiva of the *Nirvanashatkam* is beyond form, language, and metaphor. There is no accurate way to describe Shiva because all descriptions arise from the relativities of language. The best a commentator can do when discussing the transcendent is to admit that he can never describe what the transcendent "is." But he can make an effort to describe what the transcendent "is like." With this approach, the intuitive reader may draw near to one that can never be seen with the eye nor known by the mind.

Nirvanashatkam

Six Stanzas on Nirvana
by
Shankara

1

मनो बुद्ध्यहङ्कार चित्तानि नाहम्
न च श्रोत्र जिह्वे न च घ्राण नेत्र ।
न च व्योमा भूमिर्न तेजो न वायु
चिदानन्द रूपः शिवोऽहम् शिवोऽहम् ॥

mano buddhyahaṅkāra cittāni nāham
na ca śrotra jihve na ca ghrāṇa netre
na ca vyomā bhūmirna tejo na vāyu
cidānanda rūpaḥ śivo-ham śivo-ham

*I am not the mind, not the intellect, not the ego,
not the personal consciousness.
I am not the ears or tongue, nor the nose or eyes.
I am not the ether or the earth, not fire or wind.
My form is the bliss of consciousness,
I am Shiva, I am Shiva.*

The form of this verse is one which Shankara duplicates through-out the text. It will, therefore, be helpful for the reader to understand his style of presentation. Shankara, being a *jnana* yogi, a yogi of the path of wisdom, writes with two purposes: to affirm what is eternal, and to negate what is temporal. His affirmation involves correctly identifying the one, eternal, conscious Self, whom he calls Shiva. His negation dissects from the Self what is limited, temporal, and insentient. In the verses of the

Nirvanashatkam, Shankara guides the reader on a tour of creation designed to differentiate Shiva, the conscious observer, from creation, the insentient observed.

Shankara begins his work by presenting the various aspects of the limited human consciousness, and impelling the aspirant to negate identification with them. For the vast majority of aspirants, this negation will only be possible after understanding exactly how human consciousness operates.

Most of us are so identified with our bodies and minds that it is nearly impossible for us to detach our pure sentience from these vehicles of incarnation. When we deeply understand the true nature of the body and mind, however, the realization of our transcendence spontaneously arises.

The basic mechanism of human consciousness is known as the *antahkarana,* the four-fold instrument. The *antahkarana* is comprised of four components: *manas,* mind; *buddhi,* intellect; *ahamkara,* ego; and *chitta,* substratum of personal consciousness. We briefly examined the *antahkarana* in verse 7 of the *Pratyabhijna Hridayam;* here we will explore in more detail how the four components interface with each other.

The *manas,* or mind, is the aspect of consciousness which engages the external world. *Manas* absorbs information from the sensory organs and collates this input, producing a composite depiction of the material world. Its domain is limited to the realms perceivable by the five senses: the world of matter and physical phenomena.

The *buddhi,* or intellect, directs the *manas* and sense organs. The intellect commands the mind and senses in their affairs based on personal inclinations. Like an admiral at the helm of a ship, the intellect gives orders to the senses and mind. When the *buddhi* is healthy, the ship of consciousness sails with a direction and purpose. If the intellect is flawed, the individual loses his sense of spiritual reality and flounders in confusion about life's meaning and the way to fulfillment.

The *ahamkara,* or ego, is the sense of "I am me, a unique individual." It serves as the ultimate executive function over the *buddhi* and *manas.* The ego commands the *buddhi* to use its troops to go into the world and return with treasure and pleasure. When the ego is healthy, it appreciates that it is one individual amongst billions. It perceives that it must share the resources of the world if peace and harmony are to reign. When the ego is unhealthy, its selfish tendencies drive it to secure pleasure and avoid pain at any cost. It becomes self-obsessed, losing its sense of community and responsibility.

The *chitta* is the substratum of personal consciousness. The *chitta* is the soil in which the plants of ego, intellect, and mind sink their roots. As discussed in verse 7 of the *Pratyabhijna Hridayam,* the *chitta* is the home of the *samskaras,* the seeds of impulse, which form the basis of motivation for the individual.

The following example depicts how the four components of the *antakharana* work together. John the yogi walks out of his house one night and looks at the sky. His *manas* processes the sensory information provided by his eyes, and forms a picture of a black celestial ceiling containing a round, glimmering object. His *buddhi* identifies the scene and labels it "the moon in the evening sky." His *ahamkara* responds with inner dialogue akin to, "I, John the yogi, am enjoying looking at the moon." The *chitta* absorbs the experience and preserves it in the form of a *samskara.* This *samskara* of pleasure will rest in the *chitta,* and later motivate John to again look for the moon.

The second line in this verse identifies the sense organs which receive information from the world, called the *jnana indriyas,* "the senses of knowledge." These are, again, instruments belonging to the Self, Shiva. Since these instruments are not synonymous with Shiva's identity, one should practice detachment from them. The *jnana indriyas* can be used efficiently during the life span of the body without requiring undue attention.

The third line refers to the *bhutas,* "material elements," which form the structure of the external world, including one's physical body. These elements are not matter per se; they are sub-physical forces which result in the formation of matter, somewhat in the same way atoms eventually coalesce into matter. Shankara goes into detail about the formation of matter from the *bhutas* in some of his other works, such as the *Tattva Bodha*.

In this first verse, Shankara identifies how personal consciousness, the senses, and the body are separate from one's true self, Shiva. The body/mind complex is an instrument, or a vehicle, like an automobile, which is used by the self during its incarnation.

The vehicle is to be tended with care, but when its usefulness is completed it is to be disposed of like an old car ready for the junk yard. Such is the attitude towards the body held by the accomplished yogi of the *jnana* tradition.

This extreme degree of detachment can be disturbing, but it must be contemplated if one is to understand an important stream of ideas in the yogic trinity. For the advanced *jnana* yogi, Shiva—God transcendent—remains eternally beyond all creation and manifestation. God resides in heaven, not on earth, and this is why so many yogis who worship the transcendental Shiva renounce the world. For them, the world is something to grow out of, a school from which to graduate.

The *jnana* yogi does not seek to improve the world because s/he lives with a dichotomy between heaven and earth. S/he perceives heaven as a plane of reality for those whose consciousness has been absorbed in Shiva. Earth is a plane of reality for those who are absorbed in self-centered, egocentric desires.

From this point of view, the earth cannot be improved to a great extent because it is a low level of reality, designed to serve as the abode of beings who are yet to attain spiritual consciousness. This position may be difficult to accept for those concerned with issues of social justice and environmental improvement, but it remains a considerable influence in yogic thought.

The essential principal of this first verse is simply that Shiva is not the body or the mind. He is eternal bliss. Any state of consciousness other than bliss belongs to the body/mind complex, and should be eschewed in order to approach the consciousness of Shiva.

2

न च प्राणा संङो न वै पञ्च वायु
न वा सप्त धा तुर्न वा पञ्च कोषः ।
न वाक् पाणि पादम् न चोपस्थ पायु
चिदानन्द रूपः शिवोऽहम् शिवोऽहम् ॥

na ca prāṇā saṁno na vai pañcā vāyu
na vā sapta dhā turnna vā pañcā koṣaḥ
na vāk pāṇi pādam na copastha pāyu
cidānanda rāpaḥ śivo-ham śivo-ham

I am not the universal life force,
nor the five energies within the body;
Nor am I the seven basic principals, nor the five sheaths.
I am not speech or hand or feet,
not the organs of reproduction or elimination.
My form is the bliss of consciousness,
I am Shiva, I am Shiva.

According to yoga philosophy, there is one universal life force that animates all things. Called *prana* by Shankara, it is also known as *shakti* and *kundalini* in other yogic traditions. *Prana* is the power which gives life and movement to all forms of inert matter. The same *prana* causes the sun to shine and your heart to beat; the same *prana* causes the grass to grow and your food to digest. All life forms are powered by the same cosmic electricity. We are all plugged in to one divine generating system.

According to the Ayurvedic medical system, sometimes called "yoga's sister science," the universal, macrocosmic *prana* manifests as five energies within the body. These are the *pancha vayus,* or "five winds" mentioned in the first line of this verse. These "winds" are vital forces which provide for the functioning of the human body. They are the microcosmic manifestation of the macrocosmic great *prana*. Their names and functions are as follows:

Udana vayu, "rising air" — The province of this *vayu* is between the throat and the top of the head. It keeps the body upright and regulates the sense of balance. It provides for the function of speech and also contributes to processes of the brain.

Prana vayu, "vital air" — Not to be confused with the macrocosmic *prana,* the province of this *vayu* is between the throat and the navel. It is primarily responsible for respiration and the exchange of gases that take place in breathing.

Samana vayu, "unchanging air" — Residing in the region between the heart and navel, the primary function of this *vayu* is to digest food and distribute its nutrients to other parts of the body.

Vyana vayu, "diffused air" — Functions throughout the entire body via the blood vessels, lymphatic system, and the nervous system.

Apana vayu, "downward air" — Lays in the area between the navel and rectum. Its primary function is the elimination of the wastes produced during the digestion of food; it is also involved in reproduction and child delivery.

In the second line, Shankara writes of "seven basic principals." Other translators have defined these as seven "components" or "elements" involved in building matter. But considering that Shankara details the *bhutas* (essential elements) and *indriyas* (sense organs) in other verses, it seems that he must have been referring to another aspect of the manifest system. Since these bases are seven in number, it is my opinion that Shankara was making reference to the seven *chakras.*

Earlier in this book (verses 3 and 7 of the *Pratyabhijna Hridayam*) we looked at the seven *chakras* and their relation to the seven levels of the universe. There the emphasis was on the macrocosmic system. Here we will shift focus and examine in more depth the relevance of the *chakras* to human psychology.

Muladhara Chakra — Located at the base of the spine, this *chakra* is associated with the root of individual existence and the fear of egoic death. When the consciousness of an individual is influenced by this *chakra,* s/he holds the thought, "I am alive and one day I will die."

Svadhisthana Chakra — Located behind the genitals, this *chakra* is associated with reproduction and issues of pleasure. When the consciousness of an individual is influenced by this *chakra,* s/he holds the thought, "I am subject to pleasure and pain from external sources."

Manipura Chakra — Located behind the solar plexus, this *chakra* is associated with personal power and issues of security. When the consciousness of an individual is influenced by this *chakra,* s/he holds the thought, "I am in competition with others for resources and social standing."

Anahata Chakra — Located behind the center of the chest, this *chakra* is related to compassion. When the consciousness of an individual is influenced by this *chakra,* s/he holds the thought, "I am one among my equals."

Vishuddha Chakra — Located behind the throat, this *chakra* is related to higher creativity. When the consciousness of an individual is influenced by this chakra, s/he holds the thought, "I am endowed with the energies of my Creator."

Ajna Chakra — Located behind and between the eyebrows, also known as "the third eye," this *chakra* is the seat of the inner guru. When the consciousness of an individual is influenced by this *chakra,* s/he holds the thought, "I know who I am."

Sahasrara Chakra — The center located at the crown of the head, related to the attainment of enlightenment by a human being. When the consciousness of an individual is influenced by this *chakra*, s/he holds a reflection of the experience of joyous awareness felt by Shiva as "I am."

We should remember that Shankara introduces these seven levels of consciousness for the purpose of encouraging the aspirant to detach from identifying with any of the lower six. Attachment to the consciousness of any of the *chakras* results in incarnation, and Shankara urges his student to transcend all embodied existence. All forms are vehicles, and Shankara encourages the aspirant to go beyond any of the structures which bind the soul.

The *pancha kosha* of the second line are the "five sheaths" which form the total composition of a human being. These sheaths serve as a map of the physical and subtle bodies. Like the *chakras,* these sheaths are identified by Shankara to inspire the aspirant to free the self from their limitations and ascend to the limitless. The sheaths are:

Annamaya kosha, "physical body" — The gross structure comprised of physical matter.

Pranamaya kosha, "energy body" — The subtle structure comprised of primal energies that provide the physical form with life force.

Manomaya kosha, "mental body" — A vibratory structure comprised of thoughts and emotions generated by contact with the external world.

Vijnanamaya kosha, "intuitive body" — A more subtle vibratory structure comprised of intuitive energy that reflects insights about the spiritual nature underpinning all experience.

Anandamaya kosha, "bliss body" — A star-like radiance too subtle to be seen or imagined, comprised solely of a reflection of the soul.

It may seem redundant for Shankara to mention the *chakras* and sheaths, and for this author to discuss them in more detail. After all, if the whole purpose is to transcend them, shouldn't we look at manifestation as distasteful and leave it behind us on our way to God? Though Shankara's emphasis is most certainly on transcendence, we shall see in our discussion of verse 6 that this does not mean he condemns the world. Shankara simply sets before the aspirant the goal of attaining the Father of creation, not any of his gifts of creation. We might think of an investor who has the opportunity to acquire various jewels such as diamonds, rubies, or emeralds. The typical person would be overjoyed to gain such an acquisition. But Shankara is trying to inspire the aspirant with the fervor and dispassion to renounce the jewels of manifest life in order to come into the presence of the jeweler himself, Shiva.

In the previous verse, the *jnana indriyas* were discussed, detailing how the body/mind complex receives information. In the third line of this verse appears mention of the *karma indriyas,* the sense organs by which the body affects its environment. The interface between the information acquired by the *jnana indriyas* and the bodily response of the *karma indriyas* is coordinated by the *antahkarana,* the four-fold instruments of consciousness discussed in the first verse.

From the point of view of the *Nirvanashatkam,* the human body/ mind, with all its wonderful tools, is like an immense super computer. Perhaps our bodies and minds are the ultimate "personal computers!" Be that as it may, Shankara reminds us again that we are not the computer, no matter how impressive it may be, but the computer operator. Computers can process almost unlimited information; they can even construct virtual realities, but they are still creations. Go beyond all the information to be known in creation, says Shankara, and find the wisdom that is in Shiva, your Self.

3

न मे द्वेष रागौ ना मे लोभ मोहौ
मदो नैव मे नैव मात्सर्य भावः ।
न धर्मो न चार्थो न कामो न मोक्ष
चिदानन्द रूपः शिवोऽहम् शिवोऽहम् ॥

na me dveṣa rāgau nā me lobha mohau
mado naiva me naiva mātsarya bhāvaḥ
na dharmo na cārtho na kāmo na mokṣa
cidānanda rūpaḥ śivo-ham śivo-ham

I experience neither attraction nor repulsion,
nor greed or delusion,
Arrogance and jealousy are not mine.
I have no social duties, nor wealth, no desires, no liberation.
My form is the bliss of consciousness,
I am Shiva, I am Shiva.

Attraction and repulsion are two of the *kleshas,* or bondages, that Patanjali refers to in his *Yoga Sutras.* Attraction and repulsion are experiences of the individual who is tossed about by external forces. Patanjali says that attraction and repulsion arise from consciousness identifying with a body/mind complex.

There is nothing inherently problematic with incarnation. The difficulty arises when the self so strongly identifies itself with its bodily and mental vehicles that it forgets the body is only a temporary abode. Under this spell, all types of delusions and conflicts arise that jeopardize the value of incarnation. When the self maintains its position as dweller in the body, incarnation becomes a valuable asset in God's great drama of creation.

Greed and delusion are two primary forces stimulating life in the realms of ignorance. Greed prods the individual to seek what s/he wants regardless of the impact on self and others. Prompted by greed, that individual believes resources are never enough, and s/he feels compelled to seek for new experiences and acquisitions. Constant seeking without satisfaction is the earmark of what Buddhists call the consciousness of a "hungry ghost."

The delusion that Shankara refers to is of a spiritual nature. It is a confusion arising from lack of direction. For those with no spiritual vision, there is no course to guide the rivers of life. Time slips by with no sense of meaning or accomplishment. Without a spiritual context for life, even the brightest of worldly enjoyments end up as ashes in a short-lived fire.

This spiritual context is called *dharma*, which denotes a harmony in relationships and with one's environment. Worldly activities become *dharmic* when they are undertaken as part of a spiritual vision. Without this spiritual understanding, activities are generally prompted by greed and delusion, and result in further karmic bondage. With an appreciation of *dharma,* activities become offerings to God undertaken on behalf of the spiritual development of oneself and others.

The third line of this verse is significant because Shankara makes reference to the four goals of life outlined in the *Vedas*. These are social duties, prosperity, appropriate desires, and spiritual wisdom. Shankara negates all of these as his goal. To understand why Shankara would encourage the complete transcendence of all traditional social success, including *moksha* (a spiritual wisdom conducive to social betterment), it is necessary to explore one of the most difficult and misunderstood aspects of Shankara's school of non-dualism: the teaching of the world-illusion.

Shankara has elsewhere written that the Absolute [Shiva] alone is real, the world an illusion. This teaching is often troubling to aspirants for two reasons. First, it flies in the face of our experience of the reality of the world. Second, it seems to imply a nihilistic view of a world without purpose or meaning. If the world is an illusion, one might well ask, Am I also an illusion? Isn't this book an illusion? Is my suffering and search for peace illusory? If all Shankara can offer is some metaphysical testimony that denies one's daily experience, then he offers no help in the search for peace.

The *advaita,* or non-dual, teachings of the illusory nature of the world are actually simple to understand and are consistent with the findings of contemporary quantum physics. To begin with, what we human beings call "reality" is not an ontological fact, but a composite resulting from the interface of ourselves and our environment.

In his *Atma-Bodhi,* Shankara uses the example of the sky appearing blue to demonstrate how what we assume to be real is not necessarily so. The blueness of the sky is the result of the refraction of the sun's light upon the human eye, and the resulting formation of a blue image in the mind. The sky itself is actually dark, empty space. The blue sky does not have an independent reality—it results from the interaction of sky, sun, and human perceiver.

The advaitans deem the world illusory when it is seen as different from Shiva. When the aspirant awakens his wisdom-vision and finds that everything is Shiva, then no separate world exists. Creation does not disappear in an amorphous cloud; rather, it shines with the light of Shiva's presence. To the enlightened advaitan, the sky still appears blue, but s/he intuits the foundation of this phenomenon to be the eternally transcendent consciousness of Shiva. The sky is Shiva, the sunlight is Shiva, the eyes and mind are Shiva. There is no world because nothing exists but Shiva.

4

न पुण्यम् न पापम् न सौख्यम् न दुःखम्
न मन्त्रो न तीर्थम् न वेद न यज्ञः ।
अहम् भोजनम् नैव भोज्यम् न भोक्त
चिदानन्द रूपः शिवोऽहम् शिवोऽहम् ॥

na puṇyam na pāpam na saukhyam na duḥkham
na mantro na tīrtham na veda na yajñāḥ
aham bhojanam naiva bhojyam na bhoktā
cidānanda rūpaḥ śivo-ham śivo-ham

I have no virtue or vice, no pleasure or pain.
I have no mantras or places of pilgrimage,
no scriptures, no ceremonies to perform.
I am not the one who eats,
not the food that is eaten, not the act of eating.
My form is the bliss of consciousness,
I am Shiva, I am Shiva.

The religion of India during Shankara's lifetime was obsessed with proper religious and social conduct. Beginning with the *Vedas* and the *Codes of Manu*, life for the devout Hindu was rigidly structured. The orthodox Hindu observed regulations and prohibitions related to virtually every aspect of life: eating, bathing, socializing, prayer, birth, death, etc.

During Shankara's life, the brahminic, priestly class held such a strong sway over society that the general population was excluded from participation in most significant aspects of religious life. In addition, there was a widely held belief that most people were not capable of attaining enlightenment during their lifetime due to gender or social class. A woman's body was condemned as an inferior incarnation, and the non-priestly social classes were thought to not possess the intelligence or purity to understand spiritual matters. By living ethically, the priests taught, these lesser members of society could reincarnate in future births as brahmins, and then possibly attain spiritual liberation.

Because of Shankara's criticism of theism and deity worship, one of the condemnations issued against him was that his philosophy was actually "Buddhist." This may not seem terribly shocking to the contemporary reader, but during Shankara's life the brahmins were active in expelling Buddhism from India and this charge was a grave condemnation. The brahmins were so successful at attacking Buddhism that within a few centuries after Buddha's death, Buddhism was practically extinct within India. To this day, there is hardly any significant Buddhist activity within the motherland of its founder (save for the Tibetan community of exiles headed by His Holiness the Dalai Lama in Dharamsalla). Calling a philosopher a Buddhist during Shankara's time was a searing curse.

Shankara was clearly not a Buddhist, though his philosophy holds some similarities with that propounded by Gotama Buddha. The Buddha taught that all of life is suffering because pleasure and pain are like day and night of desire. Pleasure is the short-lived happiness that arises upon gaining what is desired, and pain comes from not getting the desire fulfilled. Either way, said the Buddha, selfish desire ends in suffering. In the first line of this verse, Shankara uses language shared by both yogis and Buddhists to point to a level of consciousness beyond the duality of pleasure and pain.

In the second line, Shankara casts a blow against the prescribed practices of virtually all of the Hinduism of his time. The repetition of *mantras,* going on pilgrimage, reciting scriptures, and performing ceremonies were the routes prescribed by the *Vedas* and reinforced by society as the path to heaven. But Shankara was a mystic and a yogi; he sought for more than heaven.

From the advaitan perspective, which is consistent with almost all other yogic traditions, there are many heavens and none of them are eternal. The heavenly realms exist on the astral and causal planes, and they are the abode of those who lived positive lives during their earthly incarnations. These heavens are the post-death dwellings of those whose *karma* is strong enough to earn them such a positive afterlife. But these heaven realms are still part of the cosmic space/time continuum and, as such, are temporal. Souls in these realms leave their heavenly dwelling when their positive *karma* runs down. The goal presented in this *Nirvanashatkam* is the transcendence of all *karma* and all heavenly rewards. The objective of the aspirant is to become absorbed in the transcendent Shiva, whose consciousness is ever in bliss.

The reference in the third line to the eater, the eaten, and the act of eating is fairly common in yogic writings. The import is that the entire process of eating, representing the life process itself, is cyclical. Everything is part of one circle, everything is at one time or another the eater or the eaten. Shankara again encourages the aspirant towards the bliss that remains transcendent to all temporal life and death.

At the end of the verse, Shiva again affirms his blissful nature. From an advaitan standpoint, Shiva is the true Self of all beings. Shiva is the only noun, all other beings and phenomenon are verbs, active parts of the cycle of life and transformation, of eater and eaten. Shiva is eternal.

In a common advaitan metaphor, individual consciousness is likened to air inside a jar. The air inside the jar is the same air as outside the jar. Break the jar and air unites with air. So the consciousness of an individual being is actually the consciousness of Shiva. Individual consciousness is an epi-phenomenon within the boundary of body/mind experience. When an aspirant negates identification with the body/mind complex, s/he attains realization. Instead of believing, "I am ordinary old John Smith, born on such a date," he realizes he is the foundation of all existence. He cries out: "Shivo-ham, Shivo-ham. I am Shiva, I am Shiva."

5

न मृत्युर्न सङ्का न मे जाति भेदः
पिता नैव मे नैव माता च जन्म ।
न बन्दुर्न मित्रम् गुरु नैव सिश्यम्
चिदानन्द रूपः शिवोऽहम् शिवोऽहम् ॥

na mṛtyurna saṅkā na me jāti bhedaḥ
pitā naiva me naiva mātā ca janma
na bandurna mitram guru naiva siśyam
cidānanda rūpaḥ śivo-ham śivo-ham

I do not die and I do not fear, I belong to no social class.
I have no father, I have no mother, I have never even been born.
I have no brothers nor friends, neither a guru or a disciple am I.
My form is the bliss of consciousness,
I am Shiva, I am Shiva.

This verse continues the process of negation that will reveal the transcendent Shiva underlying all temporal phenomenon. This process ultimately involves the negation of all that we would consider "external reality." Advaitans believe the idea of an individual born in a pre-existing world, then later dying, is nothing but a mental construct. This philosophy holds that the world arises in consciousness, not the other way around. The experience of dreaming is often used to highlight how a world can arise within the mind. In fact, say the advaitans, the entire world is nothing but a dream existing within the consciousness of the beholder.

In his *Viveka-Chudamani, The Crest Jewel of Discrimination,* Shankara presents his theory of how this dream state arises. He states that the Absolute (Shiva) is an undivided, absolute unity who knows only bliss. Shiva can never be sundered or limited, nor could he ever suffer. In order to explain our everyday experiences of limitation, division, and suffering, Shankara posited a phenomenon called *maya,* "the measurer." *Maya* precipitates the dream of the world.

Shankara never really explains how *maya* functions. After all, if Shiva is eternally unlimited and blissful, nothing could ever change or disturb this status. Still, Shankara acknowledges, multiplicity and suffering seem to occur, so he postulates maya as an illusory creator of an illusory dream. If this seems difficult to understand, know that Shankara has had many critics who have pointed to this weak link in his philosophy. For our purposes, the essence of Shankara's teaching in this regard is as follows: the world is a dream illusion as long as the aspirant identifies with a body/mind complex. When he awakens to his identity as Shiva, the dream is over and the illusion of a separate world ceases in Shiva's non-dual bliss.

In the *sanyasin* traditions established by Shankara, when one becomes a renunciate one renounces all family ties. S/he claims no particular family or clan, aligning instead with his guru and spiritual lineage. The third line of this verse is particularly striking, then, because the aspirant is to affirm that he has no guru, that he claims no discipleship, no lineage. This is an incredibly radical idea in the yogic tradition because of its emphasis on disciple transmission and initiatory rites.

It may be difficult for those of us conditioned by democratic principals to appreciate what it means for a yogi to claim he has no guru. The guru-disciple relationship is at the center of the yogic understanding of spiritual growth and enlightenment. This is not just the result of an ingrained sense of orthodoxy, either. It arises from the experiences of generations of sincere seers who have recognized how subtle is the spiritual path and how easy it is to mislead oneself.

In recent years, some in the west have likened the spiritual process of entangling egoic constructs to the experience undergone by a patient in psychotherapy. There are similarities to these processes, but spiritual enlightenment is of a qualitatively different nature than psychological development. Psychology is based on developing a healthy individuality, while yogic spirituality seeks an experience of complete transcendence of individuality. A healthy individuality is certain of importance for a citizen to function in society, but we must not forget that the yogic path is not so much concerned with personal betterment as it is with transcendence of the personal.

The path of spiritual growth is the most refined and subtle experience possible. Just as I would question the competency of a physician who never attended medical school but was instead self-taught, it is my personal opinion that no one who claims enlightenment without at some point coming into relationship with an authentic guru is fooling themselves. There is an old adage that comes to mind: "The one who is his own guru has a fool for a disciple."

It is obvious that Shankara is not offering this line as an affirmation to be used by aspirants. I have met too many immature aspirants who were quick to reference Shankara and other enlightened *jnana* yogis as proof they had no need of a guru. It was evident that they were fooling themselves. They could speak most eloquently about their identity beyond body and mind, about "having no guru and being no one's disciple," but how quickly they lost their temper when breakfast was a bit late! In fact, there are a number of parables in the bhakti and tantric traditions (some even using Shankara as a foil) that describe the blunders made by those aspirants who intellectually, but prematurely, attempt to claim the status of being beyond the need for a guru.

To be beyond the need for guidance is the summation of the spiritual journey. Advaitans believe realized yogis can attain unity with Shiva, yet this stage is very exalted and rare. Even Paramahansa Ramakrishna, the Great Swan himself, was reluctant to talk in these terms. He repeatedly told his followers to adopt the attitude of servant or devotee to God.

Still, Shankara reminds us in these bold verses that Shiva is our reality. We must be courageous enough to dare to breach the heresy of God-identification that cost Christ his life. Yet we must also be humble enough to recognize that our immediate identities are so insignificant and exist so briefly that the infinite universe does not even take notice of our lives. To intuit one's true Self as the Self of all existence, while at the same moment honoring our immediate limitations: such is the razor's edge the aspirant walks.

6

अहम् निर्विकल्पो निराकार रुपो
विभुत् वाच् सर्वात्र सर्वेन्द्रियाणाम् ।
न चा संगतो नैव मुक्तिर्न मेय
चिदानन्द रूपः शिवोऽहम् शिवोऽहम् ॥

aham nirvikalpo nirākāra rūpo
vibhut vāc sarvātra sarvendriyāṇām
na cā saṁgato naiva muktirnna meya
cidānanda rūpaḥ śivo-ham śivo-ham

I have no thought of identity, no form,
I exist everywhere, in everything, as all that can be perceived.
I am not detached, nor liberated from the limited.
My form is the bliss of consciousness,
I am Shiva, I am Shiva.

This verse is reminiscent of the statement made by Ramana Maharshi when he was approaching death in 1950. Some distraught followers pleaded with him, "Please, *Bhagavan,* don't leave us."

"Don't be silly," replied the *maharshi,* "Where could I go?"

It may be said there are three types of people in this world. The first, ordinary people, believe themselves to have been born into a world from which at death they will pass. They have no concern with spiritual concepts, such as bondage or liberation. They are satisfied with the few morsels of family security and moments of happiness that their *karma* allows. They have a vague sense, provided by a socially-sanctioned religion, that the after-life will be peaceful if they lead a decent and productive life.

The second type of people, the spiritual aspirants, seek to peek behind the curtain of the theater of incarnation. They seek to understand the great mystery of life and death. Bland theological explanations and religions designed for the masses do not satisfy their hunger. They seek for the direct, personal experiences which alone provide answers to life's great questions. To accomplish this goal, they undertake spiritual disciplines and study the wisdom teachings of the great mystics.

The third type of people are the realized souls. They have realized the individual soul, the *jiva,* as one in God, Shiva. The wave has merged into the ocean. Wisdom has penetrated to the very depths of existence, to the throne of Shiva, the King of Heaven. No limiting thoughts or forms are confused with the soul. Nature, other beings, even the body appear as simply phenomenon on the screen of consciousness. The dance of creation and destruction takes place through the ages while the Lord sits in the hall of eternity.

There is one additional tenet to Shankara's philosophic platform that should be addressed: his teaching on the immediacy of self-realization. Shankara, like other *jnana* yogis, holds that the aspirant already possesses that which is sought. Individual consciousness is already one with Shiva, as the wave is already one with the ocean. The aspirant need only still personal consciousness, including even thoughts about spirituality, in order to realize Shiva. Self-realization is not an experience to be attained in time. It is the eternal state, ever available in the immediate moment.

The idea of the immediacy of self-realization has its foundation in the *Upanishads,* and Shankara is its most significant historical proponent. This ancient teaching has been revitalized in the 20th century by Ramana Maharshi, Nisgardatta Maharaja, and Jiddu Krishnamurti. Shankara, Ramana Maharshi, and Nisgardatta Maharaja were *jnanis* from the alpha point of their spiritual life. Krishnamurti's development was rather different. A brief review of his life and philosophy is helpful in assessing the glories and problems of the teaching on the immediacy of self-realization.

As a young boy, Krishnamurti was playing on a beach in 1909 when he was "discovered" by Charles Ledbetter. Ledbetter, along with Annie Besant, had popularized the Theosophical Society founded by Madam Blavatsky, author of The *Secret Doctrine.* Krishnamurti was identified by Ledbetter and Besant as the World Teacher, a sort of 20th century Christ. He was groomed for this position from his youth, and his early writings are filled with references to classic theosophical experiences, such as astral visits with the Masters of Wisdom, who make up what is known as the Hierarchy, or the Great White Brotherhood.

Krishnamurti engaged in a variety of spiritual disciplines and had many spiritual and psychic experiences. Then, quite suddenly, in 1929 he renounced his position as a teacher and disowned himself from the Theosophical Society. This was a stunning move and threw the occult world of his time into turmoil. Krishnamurti spent the 56 remaining years of his life preaching a philosophy similar to that presented by Shankara in this text.

Krishnamurti called spirituality a "pathless path," and he admonished against participation in most of the significant landmarks of the Indian spiritual geography, such as meditation, ceremonies, and devotion to a *guru*. Krishnamurti engaged his followers (though he disdained being called a leader) in Socratic dialogues which he hoped would stimulate them into the immediacy of the present moment, beyond the mind and all of its conditionings.

Shankara, as we know from this text and his other writings, held views similar to those spoken by Krishnamurti some 12 centuries later. But tradition holds that Shankara actually transcended this somewhat dogmatic negativity against the path, after an experience toward the end of his life. Purportedly, Shankara was once taken so ill that he did not have the strength to climb a flight of stairs to a temple where he was scheduled to preach. A pretty young girl saw the sage and asked, "Sir, why do you lie on the ground in such a condition?"

"Can't you see?" replied the great man of wisdom. "I am ill. I have no *shakti*." (a Sanskrit term for energy or life force, as well as a synonym for *maya*).

"But Swami," smiled the girl, "all these years you have taught that *shakti/maya* is an illusion. How can an illusion cause you suffering?" And with these words the little girl showed Shankara her true from as Durga, the Divine Mother described in the *Pratyabhijna Hridayam*. Shankara then achieved full realization because his heart opened to the immanence of God, to go along with his great vision of transcendence. The story may not be entirely factual, though it might explain why Shankara, the intellectually austere philosopher and writer, would compose a number of delicate devotional poems in praise of the Goddess.

The *Nirvanashatkam* points the aspirant towards the foundation of consciousness, the transcendent Shiva. When one realizes the truth of the affirmations and negations presented in this text, one reaches the summit of *advaita*. Limited personal consciousness falls away and one exclaims in ecstasy: "Shivo-Ham, Shivo-Ham! I am Shiva! I am Shiva!"

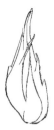

Part III

The Guru

In this section we will examine The *Hanuman Chalisa, Forty Verses Praising Hanuman,* composed by the great *bhakti* yogi Tulsi Dass in the 16th century. It is an extremely popular text with yogis who adopt either Sri Rama or Hanuman as their *Ishtadeva.* The story of Sri Rama and Hanuman is depicted in one of India's national epics, *The Ramayana,* which has been loved and revered in India for 2000 years. The *Hanuman Chalisa* narrates many of the significant events of the *Ramayana* in which Hanuman plays a key role.

The *Ramayana,* literally, "Rama's tale," tells the story of the life of Sri Rama, an incarnation of God as a human being. As a prince, the youthful Sri Rama marries the virtuous princess, Sita. Though Sri Rama is destined to become king of Ayodhya, jealousy and political intrigue result in Sita and him being banished to the forest for fourteen years. During their exile, Sita is kidnapped by the demon king Ravana. Sri Rama is assisted in his efforts to free Sita by an army of monkeys and bears led by the noble and courageous monkey, Hanuman. Sita and Sri Rama are eventually reunited, they become king and queen of Ayodhya, and their subjects live happily ever after.

The sensitive student of the *Ramayana* and the *Hanuman Chalisa* quickly comes to appreciate how brilliantly these texts use familiar symbols—kings, queens, monkeys, bears—to convey abstract teachings of yogic spirituality.

Hanuman is a unique figure, depicted as the son of a monkey mother and a divine father, the wind god. He is the symbol for the *guru,* divinity manifest in physical form. While the typical human mind is like a monkey, jumping from thought to thought, never still or content, Hanuman demonstrates how to devote the mind to God and become a peaceful and energetic partner in God's creative enterprises. Men and women who realize their own divine nature through devotion often feel the longing to share their peace and joy with suffering humanity. Such wise and compassionate ones become *gurus,* guiding others towards the realization of their own divinity.

The *Hanuman Chalisa* appears to be simply a series of verses by which the reciter offers praise to a deity outside himself. In addition to this exoteric meaning, there lays a rich symbolism and esoteric significance to the text that my commentary will reveal. The *Hanuman Chalisa* not only describes the nature of the external *guru,* it is a manual for the realization of the inner *guru* within the chamber of one's own heart. Understanding the true significance of the *Hanuman Chalisa* helps the aspirant come to a clearer perception of the roles of both *guru* and disciple in the yogic tradition.

Hanuman Chalisa

by

Tulsi Dass

श्री गुरुचरन सरोज रज निजमनु मुकुरु सुधारि ।
बरनउँ रघुवर बिमल जसु जो दायक फल चारि ॥

śrī gururcarana saroja raja
nijamanu mukuru sudhāri
baranauṁ raghuvara bimala jasu
jo dāyaka phala cāri

Polishing the mirror of my mind
with the dust of my guru's lotus feet,
I declare the eminence of the venerable best of the Raghus,
the giver of the four boons of life.

बुद्धिहीन तनु जानिके सुमिरैं पवनकुमार ।
बल बुद्धि विद्या देहु मोहिं हरहु कलेस विकार ॥

buddhihīna tanu jānike
sumirauṁ pavanakumāra
bala buddhi vidyā dehu mohiṁ
harahu kalesa vikāra

Realizing my weakness and lack of wisdom,
I pray to you, Son of the Wind,
Grant me strength, discrimination, and insight,
and remove my bondage and impurities.

These introductory verses are offered to help the aspirant cultivate a certain *bhava,* or devotional mood. The prayer to one's *guru* is a traditional opening gesture of respect and humility. Sri Rama is identified as "the best of the Raghus," the culmination of his ancestry, because an enlightened being is the culmination of the biological and cultural forces which have shaped a family lineage. He or she is the fruit of the tree of nature, whose very purpose is to bear forth those enlightened beings who can be vehicles of love in the world.

The four boons of life alluded to are: *kama,* health; *artha,* prosperity; *dharma,* harmonious relationships; and *moksha,* spiritual enlightenment. From the traditional yogic perspective, these are the riches of life resulting from righteous conduct. The spectrum of these boons reflects a beautiful and holistic view of life which encompasses all aspects of the human experience.

The second verse alludes to Hanuman as the son of the wind god, Vayu, and symbolism of Hanuman's ancestry will be discussed fully in the text. The prayer voiced at the end of this verse for insight and the removal of bondage highlight the internal focus and spiritual purpose of the *Hanuman Chalisa.* Asking for strength and determination in this context is to aid the aspirant in accelerating his spiritual development. Before beginning the recitation of the *Chalisa,* the aspirant is encouraged to seek qualities which will enable one to love God with one-pointed devotion.

1

जय हनुमान ज्ञान गुन सागर ।
जै कपीस तिहूं लोक उजागर ॥

jaya hanumāna jñāna guna sāgara
jai kapīsa tihūṁ loka ujāgara

Hail, Hanuman,
ocean of realization and virtues,
hail, master of the monkey mind,
bringing enlightenment to the three worlds.

In this first verse, the relationship between spirituality and morality is immediately introduced. Hanuman is described as a realized being and one possessing virtue. In the yogic tradition, it is understood that no one can achieve an elevated spiritual state without cultivating a high moral standard. This is not because a judgmental or vengeful deity will prevent his success, but because his own consciousness will determine at which level of reality he will abide.

A yogi with a strong character will be capable of integrating the powerful energies emanating from the higher realms. An individual of weak virtue is like a small airplane which cannot withstand the pressure of higher altitudes. It is a beautiful fact that only those whose eyes are purified of selfishness have the vision to see the gates of heaven.

Hanuman is called "master of the monkey mind," as yogic texts often compare the mind to a monkey because of its inherent tendency to chatter and remain in movement. One who can tame the monkey mind can see deeper into one's own true nature, just as one can see the bottom of a pond when it is without waves. The stilling of the mind brings realization of one's spiritual identity transcendent to the physical and mental worlds.

Many yogis still the mind while sitting in meditation and achieve the condition of *samadhi*. Some yogis can remain in this state of transcendence for days at a time and this condition of transcendence is viewed as the aim of spiritual practice in some traditions. But the *Hanuman Chalisa* gives a more developed vision of the benefit of stilling the mind and achieving *samadhi*.

In the last line of this verse, we see that one who stills the mind becomes the bringer of enlightenment. S/he does not remain sitting on the mediation blanket in a remote cave; rather, s/he brings the fruit of all efforts to his or her brothers and sisters who still linger in *avidya*, spiritual confusion. S/he becomes a spiritual adept, capable of sitting in *samadhi*, but equally attentive to the service of others. S/he becomes a *guru:* a manifestation of God in human form.

2

राम दूत अतुलित बलधामा ।
अंजनि पुत्र पवन सुत नामा ॥

rāma dūta atulita baladhāmā
aṁjani putra pavana suta nāmā

Envoy for Sri Rama,
conduit of unbridled energy,
Child of the Shining One,
called Son of the Wind.

As we saw in the introduction, Sri Rama was an incarnation of Vishnu and was Hanuman's *Ishtadeva*. Hanuman serves as an envoy of Sri Rama in the world. The *guru* serves as a link between souls bound by ignorance and the unbridled, infinite energy of the divine.

As previously mentioned, Hanuman is the child of a monkey mother, Anjani, and a divine father, the wind-god, Vayu. His birth was an interesting case of immaculate conception. One day, Anjani was walking down a forest path and Vayu was so attracted to her beauty that he flew up her skirt! Later, Anjani, like Mother Mary, was surprised to find herself pregnant without having had sexual contact with a male.

The symbolism portrayed is that spirit, God, is so attracted to the beauty of his creation that he willingly, even passionately, descends into matter. He does so in order to foster the welfare of his children and direct the process of spiritual evolution. This teaching should bring comfort to those who wonder if God is aware of our perils and plights as insignificant human beings. Krishna announced in the *Bhagavad Gita* that God incarnates on earth to restore righteousness whenever the forces of selfishness become too predominate. And Jesus taught his followers that God is aware of even the "fall of a sparrow."

God still nurtures the spark of divinity that he planted in our souls at the dawn of creation.

3

महावीर बिक्रम बजरङ्गी
कुमति निवार सुमति के सङ्गी ॥

mahāvīra bikrama bajaraṅgī
kumati nivāra sumati ke saṅgī

Great hero of immense courage,
endowed with a thunderbolt body,
dispeller of negativity,
companion of the noble

The referral to Hanuman's thunderbolt body is similar to Patanjali's mention of the *vajra,* or "adamantine" body of an accomplished yogi. To manifest God's power on the material plane, the yogi needs a nervous system capable of withstanding the constant stress inherent in physical incarnation. In addition, the aspirant who lives in modern society will need a body powerful enough to transcend the stress and negativity of daily life.

The dispeller of negativity is one who brings the light of love into situations of anger and confusion. He is the redeemer, the companion of noble souls. They hear his voice, the "still, small voice," with the ears of their intuition, within the tender chambers of their hearts. Those who participate in dispelling negativity and spreading vibrations of peace and brotherhood serve as guides and *gurus* to those imprisoned by selfish egoism. They are part of the monkey army that assists Sri Rama in his redemption of the world.

4

कंचन बरन विराज सुबेसा ।
कानन कुंडल कुंचित केसा ॥

kaṁcana barana virāja subesā
kānana kuṁḍala kuṁcita kesā

Golden radiance,
beautiful appearance,
rings are in your ears
and your hair is curly.

This verse serves two purposes. First, the depiction of Hanuman's radiance and appearance are intended to highlight divinity dwelling in physical form. The physical body of an elevated soul who is dedicated to service is a glorious vehicle of communication between heaven and earth. Most people use their bodies to strengthen their personal identity and manipulate the world to attain their petty desires.

The physical forms of the enlightened ones, though obviously consisting of material elements, are transcendent bodies. This does not mean their feet do not walk on the ground, but that their bodies have become sanctified through devotion. Their bodies become like satellite stations of the divine transmitter, broadcasting signals of love and spirituality to their families and communities.

The second purpose of this verse is to help the aspirant visualize an image of Hanuman upon which s/he can meditate. Creating a mental image is a yogic practice designed to apply the imagination for spiritual development. The imagination can be a powerful instrument, and its utility is appreciated in the Hindu and Buddhists worlds. The images formed by yogis, whether physical forms established in temples or mental images enshrined in their hearts, provide for the opportunity for *darshan.*

Darshan, literally "seeing," gives God an opportunity to manifest through a form which the devotee has created. Within the context of this text, Hanuman's physical form is to be imagined within the mind, creating an image which Hanuman can then use to communicate to his devotee.

This practice is so simple, yet so effective. Many yogis actually achieve a direct communication with their chosen deity through the experience of *darshan.*

5

हाथ बज्र औ ध्वजा बिराजै ।
काँधे मूँज जनेऊ साजै ॥

hātha bajra au dvajā birājai
kāṁdhe mūṁja janeū sājai

*Your hands hold aloft
a thunderbolt and flag,
a thread of sacred grass
adorns your shoulders.*

This verse continues the visualization begun in the previous verse. Here, Hanuman is depicted holding a thunderbolt and a flag, representing, respectively, his potency and his willingness to publicly proclaim his identity as a servant of God. The flag is a forceful reminder for the spiritual aspirant that one is not to let worldly identity supersede one's true self. There are inevitably occasions when aspirants will be forced to choose between their social *persona* and their spiritual identity. When one chooses to raise the flag of spirituality one might find that human beings, like most mammals, alienate or attack those who do not abide by the customs of the pack. The aspirant may suffer socially and economically for not fitting in, but this small sacrifice is nothing before the opportunity to serve God.

The simplicity of the sacred grass adorning Hanuman's shoulder stands in contrast to the elaborate thread worn by some boastful brahmins who parade their upper-class status. A story in the *Ramayana* depicts the value of simplicity in the vision of God. When Sita was kidnapped by the evil Ravana, she was held captive in his palace on the island of Lanka. In order to rescue his wife, Sri Rama enlisted the help of Hanuman and his army of monkey and bear allies. These mighty animals set about building a bridge to Ravana's island by throwing enormous boulders into the sea until they piled up and formed a crossing.

A small spider wished to help in Sri Rama's work, but of course she could not hurl mammoth rocks. So she did the best she could, pushing small grains of sand into the water with her tiny legs. Hanuman saw what she was doing and scolded her, telling her to move away from the great undertaking of the monkeys and bears who were tossing tons of stone. Sri Rama overheard this encounter and took Hanuman aside to correct him. He instructed Hanuman that the labor of the spider was as noble as the work of the strongest of the monkeys or bears. The success of his mission, declared Sri Rama, was dependent on the love and sincerity in which his helpers dedicated their acts.

What is of value to God is not power, or even success, but love and purity. God only asks that we do our best, for honest effort is good enough. This story also points out that no one, no matter how spiritually elevated, is perfect and above error. Only God can claim perfection.

6

शङ्कर सुवन केशरी नन्दन ।
तेज प्रताप महा जगवन्दन ॥

śaṅkara suvana keśarI nandana
teja pratāpa mahā jagavandana

*Incarnation of the Cause of Peace
and son of a mortal father,
your radiant light
is revered throughout the world.*

Shankara is a name for Shiva, God the Father, meaning "the cause of peace." One who has realized one's identity as a child of God is prepared to take his or her place among the teachers of spiritual reality. Hanuman is also identified in this verse as the son of Keshari, who was a chief in the monkey army. Keshari was Hanuman's earthly father in the same way that Joseph was the father of Jesus, though both of their progeny were conceived via immaculate conception.

The light of Hanuman is the one light revered throughout the world. Given many names through the ages, there is but One. The Vedic sages said, "Truth is one, the wise call it by many names." Krishna refers to the unity of the divine light when he remarks in the *Bhagavad Gita,* "Whatever way men may worship me, in that same way will I appear to them." Just as all humanity shares in the light of one sun, likewise does all creation share of the same creator.

Naught exists but the One, which has become many. Regardless of the form of worship undertaken when people seek for divinity, they seek the same radiant light. When Muslims bow in the direction of Allah's Mecca and Jews genuflect before Jehovah's torah, when Hindus perform *puja* to Durga and Catholics attend Mass, when Buddhists seek *nirvana* and yogis pursue the supreme Self—all strive for the same divinity.

7

विद्यावान गुनी अति चातुर ।
राम काज करिबे को आतुर ॥

vidyāvāna gunī ati cātura
rāma kāja karibe ko ātura

Full of wisdom,
virtues and compassion,
you are ever eager
to do Sri Rama's work.

In the 14th chapter of the *Bhagavad Gita,* Arjuna asks Krishna, "How am I to recognize a man of wisdom?" In other words, to whom should the aspirant turn for instruction and, even more importantly, to whom should one look as a role-model? Spiritual inspiration is not so much something that is taught, but something that is caught. This is the reason for the emphasis in the yogic tradition of the *guru* and disciple relationship. In the first part of this verse, Tulsi Dass identifies three primary characteristics possessed by a sage capable of serving as a *guru:* wisdom, virtues, and compassion.

The second half of this verse highlights the readiness and enthusiasm of the sage to be of service. The problem for most aspirants is not a matter of inspiration, it is a matter of perspiration. Laziness and lack of commitment keep aspirants from following through on their visions and manifesting their highest potential. Many aspirants have powerful experiences while sitting in meditation, but they still lack the inspiration to serve others in Sri Rama's work.

8

प्रभु चरित सुनिबे को रसिया ।
राम लषन सीता मन बसिया ॥

prabhu carita sunibe ko rasiyā
rāma laṣana sītā mana basiyā

You delight in hearing stories
of your Lord.
Ram, Lakshman, and Sita
are ever in your mind

The reference to Sri Rama, Sita, and Lakshman is intended to highlight the specific lineage from which this *Hanuman Chalisa* has sprung. Though many yogis consider the stories of Sri Rama to be allegories, there are sects that believe there exists a historical basis to the *Ramayana.*

I have personally studied in one lineage that holds that their *mantra* was first repeated by Hanuman some 10,000 years ago, and has been handed down from *guru* to disciple to this day.

9

सूक्ष्मरूप धरि सियहीं दिकावा ।
बिकट रूप धरि लङ्क जरावा ॥

sūkṣmarūpa dhari siyahīṁ dikāvā
bikaṭa rūpa dhari laṅka jarāvā

*Assuming a small form
you revealed yourself to Sita;
in an awesome form
you burned Lanka.*

These two references to Hanuman's form are allusions to a portion of the *Ramayana* in which Hanuman assists in rescuing Sita from Ravana. Hanuman discovered Sita being held captive on the island of Lanka, and he assumed the form of a small monkey so he could infiltrate her prison without being noticed by the guards.

Hanuman spoke with Sita, and reassured her of Sri Rama's abiding love and his intent to rescue her. Hanuman then allowed himself to be captured. He escaped his captors and swung through the capital of Ravana's stronghold, burning all the palaces and homes of the demons.

Symbolically, Sita represents the individual soul separated from God. The soul has come under the hold of the selfish ego (Ravana) and needs the assistance of one who is free, a *guru* (Hanuman), to regain her freedom. The *guru* reassures the soul that she is still part of God, and then destroys the strongholds of the ego, preparing for the reunion of the soul and the beloved.

10

भीमरूप धरि असुर सँहारे ।
रामचन्द्र के काज सँवारे ॥

bhīmarūpa dhari asura saṁhāre
rāmacandra ke kāja saṁvāre

Dreadful the form in which
you destroyed the demons
and accomplished the mission of Sri Rama.

As the destroyer of the demon nation, Hanuman is known as Lankabhayankaram, "the Terrifier of Lanka," which we discussed in the commentary on verse 6 in the *Pratyabhijna Hridayam*. In addition, the yogic tradition has long recognized that God appears differently to spiritually oriented individuals than he does to those clinging to selfish ego identities.

This does not mean that God decides to present himself differently based on his judgment of someone as "good" or "bad." Rather, one's perception of God results from the level of one's own consciousness. God and *guru* appear benevolent to devotees and frightening to those clinging to selfish tendencies. Those who "live in Lanka," who live in selfishness, will perceive the *guru* as frightening because they are clinging to self-centered interests out of harmony with God's will. They will feel that the *guru* is prepared to destroy their kingdom of desires and attachments. And they are right!

11

लाइ सँजीवन लखन जीयाये ।
श्री रघुवीर हरषि उर लाये ॥

lāī saṁjīvana lakhana jīyāye
śrī raghuvīra haraṣi ura lāye

By bringing the life-giving herb,
Lakshman was revived,
Sri Rama was delighted
and hugged you tenderly.

During the battle to rescue Sita, Sri Rama's brother Lakshman was apparently mortally wounded. Hanuman successfully located an herb which saved Lakshmana's life. Sri Rama was thrilled at the rescue of his brother from the clutches of death, and the *Chalisa* presents his response in this and the next two verses.

Lakshman was Sri Rama's faithful brother. He insisted on accompanying Sita and Sri Rama when they were banished to the forest for their fourteen year exile. Lakshman represents the pure mind capable of meditation and devotion. The pure mind always dwells near God, whether it is in the palace or the jungle.

12

रघुपति कीन्ही बहुत बड़ाई ।
तुमा मम प्रिय भरतहि सम भाई ॥

raghupati kīnhī bahuta barāī
tumā mama priya bharatahi sama bhāī

The Master of the Raghus
praised you:
"You are a brother,
I love you as I do Bharata."

Sri Rama is referred to as master of the Raghus, his ancestral lineage. When an enlightened being appears, the family tree has born its fruit. The essential point is not heredity, but understanding that Mother Nature works entirely on behalf of spiritual evolution. Genetic traits within an ethnicity provide a framework in which different classes of souls can partake of similar karmic circumstances. These circumstances of material nature prompt and prod the soul to transcend all limited identifications and attain realization. When this has occurred, when enlightenment arises, nature has produced her fruit.

When Sri Rama praised Hanuman as a brother he was paying him an immense compliment. No disciple dares consider himself or herself an equal, a brother or sister, with his *guru*. Spirituality is not egalitarian;

there are hierarchies of wisdom. The disciple humbly accepts the teacher as having accomplished the spiritual work toward which the disciple is striving. This is part of nature's work, to ensure that humility is one of the characteristics developed before her children attain spiritual power.

The disciple desires to serve the *guru* and to emulate the *guru's* honorable qualities. The *guru* is like a mature adult and the disciple is still a child in the ways of wisdom and devotion. Though love between parents and children is deep and beautiful, the love shared between a teacher and student on the spiritual path is even greater because of its purity and non-attachment.

13

सहस बदन तुम्हरो यश गावैं ।
अस कहि श्रीपति कङ्ठ लगावैं ॥

sahasa badan tumharo yaśa gāvaiṁ
asa kahi śrīpati kaṅtha lagāvaiṁ

*"Thousands will
sing your glory."
Saying this, the Lord of Lakshmi
took you in his embrace.*

Here Sri Rama grants Hanuman the boon of great fame. For a lesser yogi, this boon would actually be a curse, because fame is perhaps the greatest of all ego attractions. Hanuman was worthy of this grace from Sri Rama, however, because he demonstrated his ability to be of service without concern for recognition or appreciation.

This type of selfless service brings one into the embrace of God. The supreme divinity is the Lord of all created beings, worshipped by even Lakshmi, the great Goddess of Wealth. When one is able to serve the Lord from love, without concern for reward or status, one comes into intimate contact with the One who is master of masters, worshipped by beings of all rank of spiritual accomplishment.

14

सनकादिक ब्रह्मादि मुनीसा ।
नारद सारद सहित अहीसा ॥

sanakādika brahmādi munīsā
nārada sārada sahita ahīsā

Sanaka and his brother sages,
Brahma and the munis,
Narada, Sarada,
along with Shesha,

This is the first of two verses which identify significant spiritual figures who, in spite of their prowess, cannot fully expound the glory of Hanuman, the symbol of the true *guru*. Sanaka is one of four brothers who were born directly from the mind of Brahma, God as creator. They are unique in the yogic tradition because they did not need to undergo spiritual evolution. They were created by Brahma as complete and perfect. The *munis,* "silent ones," are those great seers who have silenced the agitation in their minds and are able to remain in the thunderous silence of God's presence.

Narada is a figure who appears throughout centuries of yogic writings. He travels the universe playing his vina and spreading the teachings of *bhakti* yoga, the yoga of spiritual devotion. He is also quite a trickster and is often involved in mischief of one sort or another.

Relevant to this text, Narada was involved in the circumstances which resulted in Shiva incarnating as Hanuman. One time, Shiva and Narada were attending a party in the heavenly world and Narada was very attracted to one of the goddesses who was present. Shiva, a trickster in his own right, agreed to help Narada by introducing him to her. Shiva brought the Goddess to meet Narada, but when she saw Narada she burst out laughing and walked away.

Narada was terribly embarrassed and couldn't understand why the Goddess laughed at him, until he realized that Shiva had turned him into a monkey as a practical joke. Angered, Narada cursed Shiva so that he would one day have to live as a monkey. Since the curse (and the blessing) of a sage must come true, Shiva accepted the curse as his *karma* and later incarnated as Hanuman to serve Sri Rama and resolve this destiny.

Sarada is another name for Saraswati, the Goddess of learning, music, language, and other fine arts. With all her eloquence, even she can not sufficiently praise Hanuman. Shesha is a thousand-headed snake, also known as Ananta, "the infinite," on whom Vishnu lays while dreaming the universe into existence.

15

यम कुबेर दिक्पाल जहाँते ।
कवि कोबिद कहि सके कहाँ ते ॥

yama kubera dikpāla jahāṁte
kavi kobida kahi sake kahāṁ te

Yama, Kubera,
and the guardians of the four directions,
poets, scholars—
none can describe your splendor.

Yama is the God of Death, and Kubera is the God of Wealth. Even these two, along with the learned and poetic, are at a loss to describe the greatness of a true *guru* like Hanuman. Such is the situation facing Tulsi Dass! Still, he joyously continues on for an additional 25 verses.

16

तुम उपकार सुग्रीवहिं कीन्हा ।
राम मिलाय राजपद दीन्हा ॥

tuma upakāra sugrīvahiṁ kīnhā
rāma milāya rājapada dīnhā

You rendered favor
to Sugriva,
introducing him to Sri Rama,
his throne was restored.

Hanuman was one of the ministers in the government of the monkey king, Sugriva. Sugriva had lost his kingdom to his brother Bali due to a misunderstanding. Even worse, Bali had threatened to kill Sugriva, so poor Sugriva lived in constant danger and fear. Upon meeting Sri Rama and Lakshman, Hanuman took it upon himself to introduce the two brothers to his leader. Sri Rama eventually helped Sugriva regain his throne from the unrighteous Bali.

The symbolism is that each of us is like Sugriva. We live in fear of the world and our minds are anxious over what danger might befall us or our loved ones. We have been deprived of the kingdom of inner peace, which has been taken over by the unrighteous thoughts of hurry, worry, fear, and self-doubt.

Through the grace of the *guru*, we come closer to God and eventually regain our kingdom. Hanuman's behavior in introducing Bali to Sri Rama is reflective of the way in which the *guru* helps arrange for the aspirant to be introduced to God

17

तुम्हरो मन्त्र विभीषन माना ।
लङ्केस्वर भये सब जग जाना ॥

tumharo mantra vibhīṣana mānā
laṅkesvara bhaye saba jaga jānā

Your counsel was
heeded by Vibhishana,
and he became ruler of Lanka,
as the whole world knows.

Vibhishana is a very interesting figure in the *Ramayana*. He is the brother of Ravana, the ego-demon king, but he ends up siding with Sri Rama in their great battle. From the moment that Ravana kidnapped Sita, Vibhishana encouraged his brother to return her to Sri Rama. At first he spoke to Ravana about proper conduct, but after these pleas fell on deaf ears, Vibhishana petitioned for Sita's return to her husband in order to avoid the downfall of the demon race.

Vibhishana met Hanuman after Hanuman allowed himself to be captured while visiting the imprisoned Sita. When Hanuman was brought before Ravana and his advisors, he warned the demons that Sri Rama would soon attack their stronghold and destroy them all. The demons, mighty warriors that they were, laughed hysterically at the idea that an army of mere mortal men, supported by monkeys and bears, could possibly defeat them. Only Vibhishana heard the truth behind Hanuman's warning.

Ravana was so furious when Vibhishana respected Hanuman's warning that he expelled his brother from Lanka. Vibhishana then sought protection with Sri Rama. Many of Sri Rama's monkey and bear advisors distrusted Vibhishana, thinking his plea for shelter was simply a military tactic. Once they allowed Vibhishana into their ranks, they reasoned, he could serve as a spy for his brother.

Hanuman alone advised Sri Rama to accept Vibhishana. He argued that anyone who approaches God must be accepted by the Lord. Even if the individual's motives later turn out to be inauthentic, still God must show mercy and accept everyone who approaches him. Sri Rama agreed with Hanuman and informed his commanders that it would be better for them to fail in their valiant efforts than for it to be said that Sri Rama turned away someone in his hour of need. Fortunately, Vibhishana was sincere in his desire to join ranks with Sri Rama, and after the defeat of Ravana, Vibhishana was installed as ruler of Lanka.

Vibhishana represents that part of our individuality which is related to the selfish ego, but still intuits the supremacy of God. Vibhishana must leave his homeland of physical and social identities in order to gain the audience of God. By doing so, he realizes his spiritual identity as a member of God's family. After the ego (Ravana) is defeated, the kingdom of individuality (Lanka) does not disappear, but the selfish ego is replaced by a healthy sense of individuality (Vibhishana) which serves God.

18

जुग सहस्र जोजन पर भानू ।
लील्यो ताहि मधुर फल जानू ॥

juga sahasra jojana para bhānū
līlyo tāhi madhura phala jānū

The sun is thousands
of miles away,
yet you wanted to swallow it,
considering it a sweet fruit.

When Hanuman was still an infant, he sought to quench his monkey hunger by plucking an orange piece of fruit from the sky, not realizing that it was actually the sun. Of course the entire solar system was plunged into darkness and chaos! Hanuman eventually released the sun, but his elders cursed him that he would forget he possessed such immense powers so he could not repeat this disruption. One of the traditional goals of chanting the *Hanuman Chalisa* is to remind Hanuman of his powers.

Symbolically, we are all just like Hanuman: representatives of God whose purpose is to serve as vessels for wisdom and compassion. We take birth full of power, but we lose it through lack of proper understanding and the social conditionings (curses) of our family and society. Through spiritual practices, such as chanting, we remind ourselves of who we really are and the nature of our mission in this world.

19

प्रभु मुद्रिका मेलि मुख माँहीं ।
जलधि लाँघि गये अचरज नाहीं ॥

prabhu mudrikā meli mukha māṁhīṁ
jaladhi lāṁghi gaye acaraja nāhīṁ

*Carrying the ring of the Lord
in your mouth,
you leapt over the ocean,
considering this nothing special.*

Foreshadowing Hanuman's discovery of the whereabouts of the kidnapped Sita, Sri Rama gave his ring to Hanuman. Hanuman was to present the ring to Sita as proof that he was truly sent by her husband. In order to reach Sita in Lanka, Hanuman leapt across the great expanse of ocean, carrying the ring in his mouth.

The ring represents the *guru's* authority. We find this idea also presented in the Bible, where Jesus is identified as "one who speaks with authority." When the aspirant recognizes that his *guru* knows the reality of God, s/he understands that the *guru* is a representative of God and can help the aspirant reunite with the Beloved.

From a yogic perspective, Hanuman's leap is one of the most significant events in the *Ramayana*. Hanuman flies all the way across the ocean to Lanka by empowering himself with the utterance of Sri Rama's name. Yet later in the story, Sri Rama cannot duplicate Hanuman's feat, but must build a bridge covering the expanse. In other words, God himself cannot equal the acts of his great devotees!

In the *bhakti* tradition, it is said the name of God is greater than God himself. For example, during his lifetime Sri Rama was able to grant enlightenment to only a small number of his followers. Yet *bhaktas* believe anyone can chant "Sri Rama" with love and devotion and attain enlightenment. An anecdote from the life of Tulsi Dass may shed some light on the power with which *bhakti* yogis hold the Lord's name.

It is said that Tulsi Dass had such faith in the potency of chanting God's names that he was able to heal others by blessing them with the name, "Sri Rama." Tulsi Dass taught his son the same skill based on his unshakable faith.

One day his son healed a group of lepers by holding his hands over them and saying, "Sri Rama, Sri Rama." When a group of onlookers reported this miracle to Tulsi Dass, they were amazed when his response was to hang his head and cry.

"Why do you cry, Master?" they asked, "your son has performed a great miracle and saved many from untold suffering."

"I cry," replied Tulsi Dass, "because after all of my instruction, my son has such little faith he found it necessary to repeat 'Sri Rama' more than once."

20

दुर्गम काज जगत के जेते ।
सुगम अनुग्रह तुम्हरे तेते ॥

durgama kāja jagata ke jete
sugam anugraha tumhare tete

The difficult tasks
of the world
become easy
by your grace.

There are two paths in life. On one, a person seeks to get what s/he can from the world. This path leads to frustration and discontentment because there is always more to be gotten from the world. The second path inspires a person to seeks what s/he can give to the world. This way leads to satisfaction and happiness because there is always more that one can give. To understand that one can be an instrument of service and grace in the world is the realization that makes one a member of a great, nameless fellowship which has existed throughout time. Its members belong to all religions and spiritual traditions. The hallmark of membership is simply that one has seen that grace and service are the purposes of human incarnation.

The grace of God is ever-present, like the sun shining its rays. But grace must be accepted to be a reality. Paramahansa Ramakrishna said the winds of God's grace are always blowing, but we must put up the sails of our faith. The following parable highlights the nature of faith.

A man went to a spiritual teacher who was reputed capable of performing miracles. The man asked for the boon to walk on water. The teacher wrote something on a piece of paper, sealed it in an envelope, and told the man if he carried this paper with him he would be able to walk on water. The man went to a nearby pond and, sure enough, he strolled out onto the water's surface. He was amazed! Curious, he opened the envelope and unfolded the paper to see what the teacher had written. On the paper was written: *Sri Rama.* "Sri Rama!" thought the man. "What's so great about that?" And with that doubt, he sank.

21

राम दुआरे तुम रखवारे ।
होत न आज्ञा बिनु पैसारे ॥

rāma duāre tuma rakhavāre
hota na ājñā binu paisāre

You are the guardian
of Ram's gate;
no one gains entrance
without your order.

Human beings need an intermediary, a *guru,* to learn the way which will bring them through the gates of higher consciousness, into the presence of God. The reason aspirant needs an intermediary is because their consciousness is completely bound within a net constructed by their own ideas. Only something from outside the net can deliver the message that will untie the knots which hold them imprisoned.

22

सब सुख लहैं तुम्हारी सरना ।
तुम रक्षक काहू को डरना ॥

saba sukha lahaiṁ tumhārī saranā
tuma rakṣaka kāhū ko ḍaranā

Those who take refuge in you
enjoy complete happiness,
and those whom you protect
have fear of nothing.

On first glance, this verse seems to to imply that adopting a devotional attitude towards an external deity will magically ensure that nothing untold will occur in the life of the devotee. While it is true that Hindu gods do offer protection to their devotees, it must also be understood that Hanuman symbolizes an aspect of an aspirant's own consciousness. It is the divinity within one's own consciousness which can prevent harm by undoing subconscious tendencies of self-destruction.

Within the *chitta,* the personal consciousness, lays a vast reservoir of motivational impulses called *samskaras,* "seeds" (the *Pratyabhijna Hridayam* called these impulses *vasanas* in verse 18). Some of these samskaras are conscious, but others are buried deep in the subconscious. From this level below mental awareness, these seeds sprout into powerful drives forcing an individual into activities and attitudes beyond rational control. These *samskaras* and their resultant momentum spin the wheel of *karma.* Until the *samskaras* are destroyed, the aspirant will not be able to take conscious command of his or her life.

Making this situation particularly troublesome is that many of the *samskaras* are violent and destructive. This is the result of all of the self-ish and angry impulses that parade in the typical person's consciousness during the course of a lifetime. In order to be a proper citizen, one will, of course, suppress the urge to act on these impulses. Still, the desires become implanted deep in the *chitta.* If not overcome through spiritual practice, the desires will eventually produce a behavioral response. Thus we can understand the phenomena of mild-mannered people suddenly "snapping" and engaging in violent or aberrant behavior.

When one turns with devotion and faith to the guru within and without, one comes into contact with that part of his consciousness which is not destructive. That part of the mind is entirely benevolent; it desires to love and to heal. The great spiritual teachers have overcome the destructive tendencies of their minds and have fully identified with this consciousness of benevolence.

As an aspirant overcomes the negative *samskaras* and links individual consciousness with the compassion of the *guru,* happiness becomes his or her lot, and no harm can come to them because there is no desire to harm.

23

आपन तेज सँहारो आपै ।
तीनों लोक हाँक ते काँपै ॥

āpana teja saṁhāro āpai
tīnoṁ loka hāṁka te kāṁpai

Your spiritual fire
is under your control;
the three worlds quiver at your roar.

When an individual engages in spiritual practices s/he develops an inner illumination, a visceral spiritual flame. This light can be seen and felt by those with developed spiritual vision. In Orthodox Christian iconography, it is frequently depicted as a light or halo around the heads of saints. This light is the cause of the peace that one feels in the presence of great spiritual people.

The three worlds are the physical world, the astral world, and the causal world. The physical world is the plane of matter, the astral world is the plane of heightened emotions and mental insight, and the causal world is the plane of spiritual archetypes and pure abstraction. To live in any of these realms is to be incarnate and to experience oneself as a separate entity. Hanuman's roar is the sound of union, or the destruction of the illusion of separation. This blast is terrifying for those who cling to separative existence. That which appears as tender mercy to the devoted seems terrifying to those attached to their ego.

24

भूत पिसाच निकट नहिं आवै ।
महावीर जब नाम सुनावै ॥

bhūta pisāca nikaṭa nahiṁ āvai
mahāvīra jaba nāma sunāvai

*Ghosts and low spirits
do not come near
to one who utters
the name of the Great Warrior.*

Ghosts and low spirits are those thoughts of hurry, worry, fear, and self-doubt that haunt the mind of the aspirant. One must become a spiritual warrior to banish these spooks of lower consciousness. Spiritual success does not come to the meek and mild; it is a path for the powerful! The aspirant must become a great warrior and battle these negative forces until they are destroyed. S/he must slay hurry with the sword of contentment, and destroy worry with the arrow of faith. S/he must annihilate fear with the ax of courage, and end the life of self-doubt with the mace of confidence. Victory comes to those who lift the weapons of spiritual virtue!

25

नासै रोग हरै सब पीरा ।
जपत निरन्तर हनुमत बीरा ॥

nāsai roga harai saba pīrā
japata nirantara hanumata bīrā

Sickness is cured
and pain removed
by constantly chanting
to brave Hanuman.

Sickness is a synonym for *avidya,* spiritual ignorance, which makes one forget one's true identity as a spiritual being. Pain is the result of feeling oneself separate from God. Through selfishness and bad habits, we become imprisoned by the ego and held captive to *karma.* But by developing courage we triumph over these difficulties. This takes discipline and commitment, including periods of formal spiritual practice, and an effort to constantly carry the energy of one's *guru* through spiritual practice and service to others.

26

सँकट ते हनुमान छुड़ावै ।
मन क्रम वचन ध्यान जो लावै ॥

saṁkaṭa te hanumāna chuḍāvai
mana krama vacana dhyāna jo lāvai

Hanuman disperses
the troubles
of those who hold his presence
during thought, speech, and action.

This verse echoes the message offered by all great spiritual teachers throughout history. They offer us salvation from the troubles and tribulations of egoic life. They invite us to manifest our divinity as teachers to those who still believe that pain and suffering are inescapable. The path to this liberation is through surrender. Surrender means we offer our physical, emotional, and mental vehicles to be used by God for his purpose. This surrender was called "practicing the presence of God" by the Christian mystic, Brother Lawrence. It means that we invite God into our hearts, our environments, our every experience. This technique results in our realizing that we have not actually accomplished anything new by inviting God into our lives, rather, we have simply become aware of the reality of God's omnipresence. When the light of God's love is shining everywhere we look, where can the darkness of troubles be present?

27

सब पर राम तपस्वी राजा ।
तिनके काज सकल तुम साजा ॥

saba para rāma tapasvī rājā
tinake kāja sakala tuma sājā

Transcendent to all
is the ascetic king, Sri Rama;
you are the performer
of his missions.

Sri Rama is identified in the *Ramayana* as an incarnation of Vishnu, the aspect of God that sustains creation and preserves morality and righteousness. Sri Rama portrayed Vishnu's will perfectly: he was a dutiful son, ideal student, faithful husband, noble warrior, and selfless king. Even while performing these duties and adopting various social roles, however, he never forsook his spiritual identity. Even while married and living in a palace, engaging in the varied social and political agendas his station in life entailed, he considered himself an ascetic, possessing nothing and owning nothing.

28

और मनोरथ जो कोइ लावै ।
सोइ अमित जीवन फल पावै ॥

aura manoratha jo koi lāvai
soi amita jīvana phala pāvai

Whatever longing people bring to you,
you provide them with the fruit of life.

One of the greatest dilemmas in theistic traditions concerns petitionary prayer. When the devotee raises a prayer to God, does God answer? Why do the answers seem inconsistent? Sometimes the non-believer seems to have his wishes granted, by luck or by fate, before the faithful receives the answer from God. What is going on?

To begin with, the materialistic person is entirely bound by his or her own *karma*. Whatever one receives is one's due. If good comes, by chance or by volition, it is a withdrawal from the balance of one's positive *karma*. The average person has neither the spiritual potency nor the direct connection with forces capable of interceding on his or her behalf that would permit one to experience much outside of the corral of one's karmic lot.

The mature aspirant does not engage in petitionary prayer. S/he understands that God is already aware of the situation and knows, better than s/he, what is for the greatest good. When an immature aspirant asks for something from God, God will grant the request only for the purpose of advancing spiritual development. When the faithful pray, God always answers. The answer, however, as the following story reveals, does not always come in the imagined form.

Once Shiva and his spouse Parvati were walking along the earth to see how things were going. A wealthy man saw them and invited them into his home. He told Shiva he would prepare the greatest of feasts and comforts, if only Shiva would wait patiently until he finished balancing his accounts. Shiva and Parvati waited until the busy man completed his tasks, after which he did fix them a fine meal in luxurious surroundings. As the divine couple prepared to depart, the merchant asked Shiva to please reward him for his hospitality.

Shiva said, "I grant that you become ten times as wealthy as you are now."

The merchant was overjoyed.

As they continued on their way, they were approached by a poor farmer who brought them into his humble home. He dropped all other responsibilities and prepared for them the finest he had to offer—a slice of bread and a glass of fresh milk from his only cow.

Shiva and Parvati enjoyed the farmer's hospitality, and when they were preparing to leave the farmer asked Shiva if he might consider rewarding him for opening his home.

Shiva responded, "I grant that your cow dies." The man felt crushed.

Soon after leaving the earth, Parvati confronted Shiva, "My dear husband, I don't understand you! The wealthy man was so preoccupied with his wealth he had the nerve to keep you waiting while he counted his gold. Still, to him you grant greater wealth. The poor man dropped everything to attend to you, yet you ended his only source of income. Whatever were you thinking?"

"Well," responded Shiva, "since the rich man was so absorbed in his wealth, I actually cursed him with more wealth. He will become more and more involved in his finances and become further removed from the divine spirit.

"The poor man was filled with devotion but still believed his income came from the cow, not from me through the cow. To help correct his misunderstanding, I removed the cause of his illusion. In fact, I see the poor man has broken free from his last remaining impediment and is now ready to join us.

"Set another seat at the dinner table, Parvati, we're having a guest tonight!"

29

चारों युग परताप तुम्हारा ।
है परसिद्ध जगत उजियारा ॥

cāroṁ yuga paratāpa tumhārā
hai parasiddha jagata ujiyārā

*Your radiance is present
in all four ages,
and your ability
draws the world's attention.*

The four ages refer to the yogic cosmological cycle. They are:

1. *Satya Yuga* — The Golden Age, when truth and morality are at their highest.

2. *Treta Yuga* —The Silver Age, when truth and morality are still the primary principals of life.

3. *Dvapara Yuga*—The Bronze Age, when truth and morality begin to decline.

4. *Kali Yuga*—The Iron Age, when truth and morality are minimal principals in life.

The four *yugas* revolve in an eternal cycle. The *guru* principal, the spirit of guidance, is present in all ages, regardless of the moral standard of humanity at any period of history. In fact, some devotional cults believe more spiritual progress can be made during the *Kali Yuga* than any other "easier" age because God so appreciates spiritual effort made under such difficult circumstances.

30

साधु सन्त के तुम रखवारे ।
असुर निकनदन राम दुलारे ॥

sādhu santa ke tuma rakhavāre
asura nikandana rāma dulāre

You are the guardian
of aspirants and saints;
beloved of Sri Rama,
you destroy the forces of discord.

One of the great strengths of deity worship in Hinduism and Buddhism is the recognition that the manifest deity has two functions, one creative and the other destructive. Fierce deities such as Rudra and Kali display fire, swords, and other weapons to symbolize the destructive forces of *dharma*. At the same time, they also express symbols of gentleness that promise to nurture the devotee. The *guru* also shares in this two-fold function: supporting those energies which further spiritual development, and vitiating those energies which attempt to retard this evolution.

31

अष्ट सिद्धि नौनिधि के दाता ।
अस बर दीन जानकी माता ॥

aṣṭa siddhi naunidhi ke dātā
asa bara dīna jānakī mātā

You bestow
the eight powers and the nine treasures;
such was the boon
granted you by Mother Janaki.

Sita is here identified as daughter of the great King Janaka. Sita's birth was miraculous, as King Janaka found her while plowing the ground to prepare it for a sacrificial ceremony. Sita, literally "the furrow-born," was given to the world by the land; she is one with Mother Earth.

The boon received by Hanuman was the eight *siddhis*, or yogic powers, and the nine treasures of devotion. The eight *siddhis* are:

1. *animan,* "atomization" — the ability to become infinitely small
2. *mahiman,* "magnification"—the ability to become infinitely large
3. *laghiman,* "levitation"—the ability to overcome gravity
4. *prapti,* "extension"— the ability to reach anywhere
5. *prakamya,* "irresistible will"—the ability to overcome the properties
   of material elements
6. *vashitva,* "mastery"—dominion over any aspect of creation
7. *ishitritva,* "lordship"—mastery over nature
8. *kama-avasayitva,* "fulfillment of desires"—the ability to manifest all
   desires

Many believe these powers are to be understood literally. Others say these powers are to be understood symbolically as representations of the power of devotion to overcome the pull of selfish desires. Regardless, any aspirant who faithfully performs the spiritual disciplines is certain to gain a potency and vitality that seem miraculous compared to ordinary people.

The nine treasures referred to are the traditional forms of devotion. They are:

1. *sravana*— enjoying listening to God's glory
2. *kirtana*— enjoying chanting or singing
3. *smarana*—remembering God at all times
4. *padsevana*—a feeling of always serving at God's feet
5. *archana*—enjoying worship
6. *vandana*—enjoying prayer
7. *dasyam*—enjoying being a servant of God
8. *sakhyam*—enjoying a feeling of friendship with God
9. *atmanivedan*—enjoying knowing the Self as God

These treasures are the nine forms of real wealth, that which moth and dust cannot corrupt. To the one who has these treasures, nothing in the world can compare. The accomplished devotee enjoys spiritual prosperity, privilege and power that no king can imagine.

32

राम रसायन तुम्हरे पासा ।
सदा रहौ रघुपति के दासा ॥

rāma rasāyana tumhare pāsā
sadā rahau raghupati ke dāsā

You enjoy the nectar of devotion
to Sri Rama,
and you are forever
his servant.

This verse points to a significant distinction between *bhakti* yoga, the yoga of devotion, and almost all other Eastern spiritual systems. In the other traditions—such as Patanjali's *raja* yoga, Vedanta, and most schools of Buddhism—the goal of the spiritual path is to become united with the Absolute. In *raja* yoga this is called "establishment in the *Purusha*," in Vedanta it is known as "merging in Brahman" and in Buddhism it is "attaining *nirvana*." Regardless of terminology, the experience sought is the individual merging into the universal, like a drop of water becoming lost in the sea.

In the *bhakti* schools, an aspirant does not wish to merge into God, s/he wishes to continuously enjoy the delight of relationship with God. S/he wishes to enjoy the taste of sugar, not become sugar. In the *Narada Bhakti Sutras*, there are eleven different types of relationships described between the aspirant/lover and God/Beloved. Hanuman is considered the foremost ideal of the yogis who have adopted the attitude of servant. Hanuman is absorbed in his devotion for Sri Rama, and he demonstrates this love through constant service. It is said Hanuman appears whenever Sri Rama's name is chanted with love and devotion, and he has vowed that as long as Sri Rama's name is chanted he will remain present on the earth to serve his master and inspire devotees.

33

तुम्हरे भजन राम को पावै ।
जनम जनम के दुःख बिसरावै ॥

tumhare bhajana rāma ko pāvai
janama janama ke duḥkha bisarāvai

Through singing your praises
one comes to Sri Rama,
and finishes the painful cycles
of karmic existence.

It is difficult to convey to those engaged in austerities how delightful, how beautiful, and how effective are devotional practices. Simply through chanting the names of God with love and devotion one can come into the presence of God himself. This is not poetic fancy; it is the experience of generations of devotees who have realized God through love. Papa Ramdas, a 20th century yogi who wandered all over India in a frenzy of God intoxication, described the nature of singing the praises of God in this way:

> "Thy glorious name is sweetness itself, bliss itself, truth itself, love itself, knowledge itself, light itself— imperishable, above and beyond everything. Thy name is the goal of all desires; it is the source of all happiness, the end and aim of all existence."*

Eastern spiritual systems are often criticized in the West for their supposed "pessimistic" outlook, with their emphasis on the prevalence of suffering. But the problem does not belong with the Eastern seers; the problem is in the minds of the critics.

With all the comforts of modern life, it is often difficult to perceive that life without a spiritual orientation is completely pervaded with suffering.

* Swami Ramdas, *At the Feet of God,* (Kerala, India: Anandashram) 1986.

In our society, it is so easy to lose oneself in superficial distractions, conveniences, and pleasures, that the deeper pain residing in our hearts stays repressed. But life without spiritual direction really is nothing more than a constant struggle to try to secure what one wants and avoid what one is afraid of. It is a whirlwind of activity without a unifying center, a battlefield of desires and conflicts triggered by external events and uncontrollable moods. Fear and anxiety permeate everything and every relationship, and this fear drives one to vainly seek security in that which can never produce peace.

The great sages taught the suffering inherent in non-spiritual life to alert us to the hopelessness of ever finding happiness in limitation. As spiritual beings, we can never find peace in limited, material objects. As eternal beings, we can never find lasting joy in finite experiences. And as children of the Lord of Love, we can never find love in relationships based on insecurity and lack. This may sound depressing to the ego-attached mind, but it is the "good news" proclaimed by every gospel of authentic spiritual liberation.

34

अन्तकाल रघुपति पुर जाई ।
जहाँ जन्म हरिभक्त कहाई ॥

antakāla raghupati pura jā-ī
jahāṁ janma haribhakta kahā-ī

*Upon death your devotee
goes to the abode of Sri Rama,
and will take rebirth
devoted to God.*

It might be said that religion is humanity's response to the mystery of death. In most Eastern spiritual traditions, reincarnation of some form is considered one of the two principals of reality. The other principal is *karma,* the law of cause and effect. The yogic tradition believes that one's present incarnation is determined by previous acts and that future incarnations will be determined by our present acts. The wheel of *karma* turns.

Karma is spoken of in disparaging terms in some Eastern schools as a type of tortuous wheel upon which we spin, with our only hope of comfort being to overcome the insistent impulses of nature which drives *karma.* The *bhakti* schools, represented by this *Chalisa* teachings, do not share this same discouragement.

Since the primary impulse for creation comes from God, everything, including *karma*, is beautiful. Human acts can distort the beauty of God's infinite energy, but only temporarily. For *karma* is not so much of a prison sentence as it is a series of teachings designed to help God's children learn how to manifest divinity in the world. Just as a person in a worldly career needs to develop skills which will ensure success on the job, similarly the soul learns the skills of wisdom, compassion, forgiveness, and humor which will help him or her function as God's representative.

The devotee does not seek to escape from continued incarnations, s/he simply desires to spend time in the company of God. Whether its called "heaven" or "the abode of Ram," these labels refer to the same plane of experience. There are limitless experiences to be had in heaven, and each devotee will be drawn to those which most attract him or her. After the stay in the heavenly realms, one's compassion will inspire one to return to the worlds of suffering in order to serve the brothers and sisters still stuck in feelings of separation.

35

और देवता चित्त न धरहिं ।
हनुमत सेइ सर्व सुख करई ॥

aura devatā citta na dharahi
hanumata se-i sarva sukha kara-ī

Worship need not be given
to any other deity;
service to Hanuman
brings complete happiness.

Statements that seem to give precedence to one spiritual figure over another must be understood properly if an aspirant is to attain vision of the universal spiritual tradition, the timeless wisdom. I once asked Swami Satyananda Saraswati about a statement similar to the one above. "Since so many spiritual writings claim superiority for their deity, which one is the best?" After all, I figured I might as well align myself with whatever figure could really deliver the goods! Why hang out with the minor leaguers if I could go right to the big leagues?

Swamiji laughed when I asked my question and responded, "They all say they are the best."

I obviously still looked confused, so he continued, "This is to inspire your devotion. Whichever form is most attractive to you, that is the best for you."

Honor God in heaven by worshipping whichever of his prophets and saints seems to most deeply touch your heart, and honor God on earth by serving all of his children to the best of your ability. What could be simpler?

36

संकट कटै मिटै सब पीरा ।
जो सुमिरै हनुमत बलबिरा ॥

saṁkaṭa kaṭai miṭai saba pīrā
jo sumirai hanumata balabīrā

Problems are abolished
and pain ceases
for the one who treasures the thought
of the warrior Hanuman.

As we saw in the introductory verses, the yogic tradition postulates four great gifts in life: *kama,* good health; *artha,* prosperity; *dharma,* harmonious relationships; and *moksha,* spiritual enlightenment. A complete life will be full of these gifts of God. Furthermore, the process of receiving these gifts is actually very simple: purify the mind of resistance to God's grace.

As discussed in verse 22, all pain arises from impulses that reside in the unconscious as *samskaras,* or tendencies. These *samskaras* drive an individual to pursue suffering. Responsibility demands the spiritual aspirant acknowledge the unconscious attraction to suffering and resistance to grace. This is why a true *guru* requires disciples to take full responsibility for their lives.

When an aspirant accepts responsibility for his or her life, the principal of *kripa* is revealed. The sanskrit term *kripa* is a compound of *kri,* action, and pa, results. Swami Satyananda Saraswati explains that *kripa* means "what you do is what you get." We reap nothing in our lives that we did not sow. An honest aspirant will acknowledge that everything in his life is the result of his actions, speech, and thoughts. Responsibility is one of the hallmarks of authentic spirituality.

37

जै जै जै हनुमान गुसाईं ।
कृपा करहु गुरुदेव की नाईं ॥

jai jai jai hanumāna gusāī
kṛpā karahu gurudeva kī nāī

Hail, Hail, Hail,
Lord Hanuman,
shower thy grace,
beloved guru.

Hanuman is referred to as the "beloved guru," a term greatly misunderstood in the West. In America we talk about financial *gurus* and computer *gurus,* but in the yogic tradition the term *guru* is reserved for one of great spiritual mastery. A true *guru* is not only enlightened, but understands the spiritual path so well that he or she is capable of guiding others to enlightenment.

Regardless of how great the *guru,* the aspirant must still complete his or her own spiritual education. Baba Hari Dass said about his work as a *guru,* "I can cook for you, but you have to eat for yourself."

The relationship between *guru* and disciple is the most intimate of all human relationships. It is built on good will, trust, and respect. The *guru* exhibits good will in sharing teachings with disciples, a sharing which is of no particular benefit to the *guru.* The *guru's* only reward is seeing the disciple develop. Just as a rich man has no financial needs of his own but may choose to help one of less wealth, so might a *guru* deem to assist an aspirant.

The disciple demonstrates trust by following the directives of the *guru.* The disciple humbly admits that s/he is like a seedling that needs help to grow into spiritual maturity. In every field of specialized knowledge—medicine, technology, and agriculture, for instance—an individual will apprentice with a master for a long period in order to also become a master. Spiritual mastery is no different.

Respect must be a two-way street between *guru* and disciple. The *guru* must never oppress the disciple, and the disciple must honor the greater wisdom of the teacher. The *guru* is one who knows who s/he is and what is his or her purpose. The disciple is one who is approaching this insight and is humble enough to learn from one of greater achievement.

38

जो सतबार पाठ कर कोई ।
छुटहि बंदि महासुख होई ॥

jo satabāra pāṭha kara koī
chūṭahi baṁdi mahāsukha hoī

One who recites these verses
one hundred times
becomes freed of bondage
and attains supreme happiness.

It cannot be emphasized too strongly how much the devotional schools of yoga value the recitation of God's names and qualities.

The *bhakti* schools recommend repeating holy names with love and devotion as the quickest way to God realization. This practice brings about freedom from the bondages of hurry, worry, fear, and self-doubt, providing a clear vision of life lived in supreme happiness.

The suggestion here that reciting the *Chalisa* one hundred times will bring about this result seems, at first glance, to suggest a magical charm or a business contract. To the cynical mind, it appears unlikely that repeating these verses a certain number of times, or any number of times for that matter, can somehow produce the glory of higher consciousness. All I can say to the skeptic is: try it!

I don't know if there is something inherent in the *Chalisa* itself that provides this promised result, or if the happiness arises from the completion of a spiritual vow, or from longing for God deeply enough to recite the *Chalisa* a hundred times. What I do know is that the *Chalisa* delivers on its promise.

If an aspirant recites the *Chalisa* a hundred times s/he will be shown the view from the mountain top. How high up the mountain the aspirant will ascend depends on the sincerity of the chanting. How long the aspirant will be permitted to stay in that state will depend on how prepared s/he is to maintain the high degree of *shakti* present in that rarefied atmosphere.

Most aspirants have a peak experience followed by a gradual let-down, with consciousness stabilizing at a more familiar level. To maintain an elevated condition, continued spiritual work is required.

39

जो यह पढ़ै हनुमान चालीसा ।
होइ सिद्धि साखी गौरीसा ॥

jo yah paḍhai hanumān cālīsā
hoi siddhi sākhī gaurīsā

*One who recites
this Hanuman Chalisa
attains perfection
in the eyes of Lord Shiva.*

This verse amplifies the point made in the previous verse regarding the efficacy of chanting as a spiritual discipline, and it introduces the figure of Lord Shiva. In this context, Shiva is the archetypal yogi and is considered the first *guru* of all yogic lineages.

Shiva is traditionally depicted in two forms which show how polar opposites are mutually inclusive aspects of the totality of God. Shiva is often depicted in eternal meditation atop the snows of Mt. Kailash. Ever in *samadhi,* meditative trance, he never stirs from his internal bliss. The universe comes and goes while Shiva sits as the eternal silent witness of the cycles of creation and destruction. In another form, Shiva is Nataraja, Lord of the Dance, the cosmic dancer from whom all creation arises and to whom it will eventually return. As Nataraja, Shiva is incessantly in motion, never resting from the acts of creation and destruction.

When one attains perfection in the vision of Lord Shiva, one has seen the truth about the paradoxical nature of God. Ever still, yet ever in movement, God looks at himself through the loving eyes of his devotees. Immanent in every atom, yet forever transcendent to all that changes, God's nature is a beautiful, sublime mystery that cannot be captured by the senses or by the thinking mind. This divine puzzle cannot be understood by the rational intellect, but it can be felt in the loving heart. God is the dialectic fulcrum upon which all opposites are resolved. By chanting the *Chalisa* with love and devotion, one attains this highest of visions.

40

तुलसीदास सदा हरि चेरा ।
कीजै नाथ हृदय महँ डेरा ॥

tulasīdāsa sadā hari cerā
kījai nātha hṛdaya mahaṁ ḍerā

Tulsi Dass is at the feet
of the Lord, praying,
"Lord, dwell always in my heart."

After Sita and Sri Rama had been reunited, Sri Rama was so immensely grateful for Hanuman's service that he reached out to give Hanuman a hug. But Hanuman pulled back! Why would this devoted lover possibly withdraw from the embrace of his beloved? Because God was drawing Hanuman into himself, and a devotee does not want to become one with God.

A devotee does not want the experience of union; s/he does not want enlightenment, s/he does not want liberation, s/he does not want to go to heaven! No, such a devotee wants to remain slightly separate from God so s/he can enjoy a relationship with the Beloved—a relationship in which the devotee can love, honor, cherish, and serve for all time.

Such is this prayer of Tulsi Dass, that he seeks not for enlightenment or yogic powers, nor any of the benefits that are his due as an accomplished yogi. He only wants to feel God in his heart. Such is the honeyed message of the *Hanuman Chalisa.*

Closing Prayer

पवन तनय संकट हरन
मङ्गल मूरति रूप ।
राम लषन सीता सहित
हृदय बसहु सुर भूप ॥

pavana tanaya saṅkaṭa harana
maṅgala mūrati rūpa
rāma laṣana sītā sahita
hṛdaya basahu sura bhūpa

Son of the wind, remover of troubles,
embodiment of auspiciousness,
dwell in my heart, O' Supreme Immortal,
aside Rama, Lakshman, and Sita.

Near the end of the *Ramayana,* Sita and Sri Rama had been reunited and assumed rulership over the good people of Ayodhya. Sri Rama wanted to repay Hanuman for his devotion and one-pointed dedication, so he offered Hanuman anything he would like.

Keep in mind, now, that Hanuman realizes that Sri Rama is God. Hanuman understands that anything he asks for will be his. For most of us, this would be a dream come true. We would ask God for something, maybe a few things, to help us get along in the world. Perhaps we would ask for good health, a bit of prosperity, possibly even greater spiritual development. Maybe we would even ask God to bring about some great positive change in the world: an end to war, a cure for cancer, a healing of the environment.

But Hanuman just shrugged his shoulders. "I don't want anything," he said. "I did it because I am your friend."

When Hanuman whispered his words of friendship in such a sweet, honest, and humble way, Sri Rama was overwhelmed by the purity of this monkey's love. Reaching over, he drew Hanuman close and held him in his arms. This embrace Hanuman could not resist. Lover and Beloved became one.

This divine hug represents the eternal completion that echoes throughout all time. The longing for this embrace is what has brought you, dear reader, to this book, to this very moment. The great Sufi mystic, Jelaluddin Rumi, said that on the path to the Beloved it is longing that does all the work. Allow the yearning in your soul to keep the fire of love for God alive and ablaze. Let it burn throughout your body and heart, scorching all negativities. Let it be the torch by which you find your way onto your spiritual path. Let it light your footsteps, and let it be the gentle glow by which you recognize the face of your eternal Beloved.

Jai Hanuman!   Jai Sita Rama!

Glossary

advaita — non-dualism

ahamkara — ego

antahkarana — four-fold inner instrument

artha — prosperity

asana — physical postures

aum — primal vibration

avidya — spiritual ignorance

ayurveda — medical system

Bhagavad Gita — yogic text

bhakti — spiritual devotion

bhava — devotional mood

bhuta — material element

buddhi — intellect, intuition

chakra — energy center

chitta — substratum of individual consciousness

darshan — seeing

dharma — harmonious relationships

gunas — qualities

guru — spiritual teacher

Indra — God of heaven (enlightened perception)

Istadeva — chosen deity

Jesus Christ — a great sage

jiva — the individual soul

jiva-mukti — liberated while incarnated

jnana — wisdom

jnana indriyas — receptive sensory organs

Kali — Goddess Kali

kama — health, literally "pleasure"

karma — cause & effect

karma indriyas — active sensory organs

kancuka — coverings

klesha — affliction, bondage

Glossary

kosha — sheath
kripa — grace
kundalini — energy of Goddess
lankabhayankaram — Terrifier of Lanka (a/k/a Hanuman)
loka — level of reality
manas — lower mind
maya — the measurer
moksha — liberation, spiritual enlightenment
munis — the silent ones
nivritti — absorption
nirvana — the bliss of freedom
Patanjali — a great sage
prana — life force
pratyabhijna — Self-realization
pravritti — manifestation
puja — ritual
purusha — pure consciousness
prakriti — the matrix of form
ramlila — play of God
samadhi — absorption of consciousness
samskara — seed, tendency, impulse
sannyasin — renunciate
shakti — energy
shanti — peace
siddhi — power
sushumna — energy channel in the subtle body
upaya — a meditative technique
vasanas — seeds, samskaras, impulses
vayu — wind
Vedas — Hindu Scriptures
vikalpa — impulse
yajna — sacrifice, offering
yuga — cosmologic age

Index

About the Author

Prem Prakash was born in the United States and spent the first fifteen years of his life like most young men of his culture—absorbed in matters pertaining to sports and sex. With the grace and guidance of his gurus he was awakened to yoga and processes of developing wisdom and compassion.

He owes an unpayable debt for the blessings and instruction of Maharaji Neem Karoli Baba, Hari Dass Baba, Babaji Maharaj, Jesus, Vijayeswari Devi Sri Karunamayi Ma, Sri Anandi Ma, Shree Maa and Swami Satyananda Saraswati, Papa Ramdas and Mother Krishnabai, Sri Shiva Bala Yogi Maharaj, Ram Prakash, and Venerable Dhyani Ywahoo.

He is the author of *The Yoga of Spiritual Devotion* (Inner Tradition International) as well as *Three Paths of Devotion* (Yes International Publishers). His writings on yoga have also appeared in a variety of publications in the United States and Europe.

Prem Prakash lives at the Kailash Ashram in Middlebury, Vermont where he serves as co-director of the Green Mountain School of Yoga. For information on the Green Mountain School of Yoga write:

Green Mountain School of Yoga
40 Court Street #3-216
Middlebury, VT 05753

Green Mountain School of Yoga web site:
http://homepage.mac.com/ppkgmsy/gmsy.html

Yes International Publishers

Yes International Publishers is the publishing arm of the Institute of the Himalayan Tradition. It offers books and tapes in wellness, yoga, leadership, mysticism, spirituality and accessories for practice.

BY JUSTIN O'BRIEN, PH.D. (SWAMI JAIDEV BHARATI)
Walking with a Himalayan Master: An American's Odyssey
The Wellness Tree: The Dynamic Program for Creating Optimal Wellness
A Meeting of Mystic Paths: Christianity and Yoga
Running and Breathing
Mirrors for Men

BY CHARLES BATES
Pigs Eat Wolves: Going into Partnership with Your Dark Side
Ransoming the Mind: Integration of Yoga and Modern Therapy
Mirrors for Men

BY THERESA KING
The Spiral Path: Explorations into Women's Spirituality
The Divine Mosaic: Women's Images of the Sacred Other

BY SWAMI VEDA BHARATI
The Light of Ten Thousand Suns
Subtler than the Subtle: The Upanishad of the White Horse

BY LINDA JOHNSEN
The Living Goddess: Reclaiming the Tradition of Mother of the Universe
Daughters of the Goddess: The Women Saints of India

BY OTHERS
Circle of Mysteries: The Women's Rosary Book by Christin Lore Weber
Soulfire: Love Poems in Black & Gold by Alla Renee Bozarth
The Yogi: Portraits of Swami Vishnudevananda by Gopala Krishna
Streams from the Sacred River by Mary Pinney Erickson & Betty Kling
Mirrors for Women by Cheryl Wall
Three Paths of Devotion by Prem Prakash

Call our Saint Paul, MN office for a complete catalog:
651-645-6808
For orders only: 1-800-431-1579
www.yespublishers.com

About the Institute of the Himalayan Tradition

The Institute of the Himalayan Tradition is a non-profit organization for study and sharing, for education and community.

It offers residential programs, classes, workshops, conferences, biofeedback, and retreats in holistic transformative training that touch daily lives from the mundane to the sacred, from business to mythology. These classes are taught and facilitated by experienced teachers who have, in turn, been taught by others, and they by others, in a direct line of spiritual teachers reaching back five thousand years. The rishi who brought these teachings to the United States in 1969 is Sri Swami Rama of the Himalayas.

The Institute offers six teacher training programs in hatha yoga and meditation. Our hatha yoga programs are registered by the Yoga Alliance in both the 200 and 500 hour requirements, ensuring certification for graduates.

An annual yoga conference is held each summer bringing international speakers, teachers, and mystics to share their wisdom and skills.

The Institute of the Himalayan Tradition investigates the essence of spirituality without the necessity for any particular dogma or doctrine. The core of all spiritual teachings of IHT is yoga meditation.

Private consultations in wellness, yoga, leadership, and spirituality are available with the teachers.

Call for information and class schedule:
651-645-1291
web site at www.ihtyoga.org.